Female Fitness;

Build the Sexy Body, The Ultimate 10 Week Weight Training, Cardio and Yoga Workout, 16:8 Fasting Diet for Increased Fat loss, Workout For Models,
Intermittent Fasting Workout, 50 Meals BONUS to Look Great, Building A Female Fitness Model Physique,

By

M Laurence

Table of Contents

1. **<u>Introduction</u>**

I want to thank you for purchasing my book "How To Build Your Best Body; The Ultimate 10 Week Weight Training, Cardio and Yoga Workout"

Having written a number of books on fitness for men and women, from HIIT workouts for MMA to weight training for Rugby body's to various books on women wanting to get into the modelling industry I wanted to take things up to a whole new level.

This book is specifically for woman who want to transform their physique. I wanted to take from the best of my books, include new information and create a total body workout combining cardio, weight training and yoga.

Whether you want to get into modelling, social media fitness, or simply want to tone up and lose fat this regime will power you towards that goal. The business of Female Fitness Modelling is a highly lucrative industry - and competitive. Actual modelling for work can cover a wide variety of jobs once you are within the industry. It's not all about catwalk modelling, it can cover a very wide arc from commercial modelling to just having a very large following on social media. Commercial modelling is probably the easiest to get into in that it covers anything from fitness model shoots to clothing, to fitness and lifestyle shoots for furniture and cars. Also the brands you can work for can range from your local gym to global companies and the money involved can be a few hundred dollars/pounds for a few hours work to thousands for a well-known make. Not only that you can even work abroad in multiple countries with expenses fully covered.

The other side of modelling is being a social media model/fitness personality. Many of my friends and clients have become experts on looking great on social media, giving out lots of useful info and tips. With this brings fans and sponsors and they earn great money without even competing or going to a casting.

So what is the key attribute of a female fitness model? They epitomize athleticism. In a word - it's all about aesthetics - visually pleasing physiques - strong legs, svelte arms, toned chest, lean back all tapering to and perhaps the most important - a tight taut flat stomach. It's leanness.

How does this book help?

This book will get you lean by combining a varied and challenging 10 week training regime, with a healthy diet plan and the secret ingredient - Intermittent Fasting. These three core elements combine to create a turbo-charged workout plan geared to burning fat and toning muscle.

However if you feel like you are not toning up and losing fat fast enough, don't get discouraged. This is not an overnight solution, and it will take time. Your body will take time to adapt to the new fitness routines. This is completely normal. To start with you'll probably find it quiet challenging. You may also want to give up after 3 days. The intermittent fasting diet might be difficult at first and initially your body will wonder what on earth is going on. You'll be compressing your eating times and it will be tricky. This shock is completely normal. The key to succeeding is to focus on why you're doing this. Whether it's for a new career or not, more importantly it is for you. To change we must endure hardship. We must persevere. If you are really struggling with the fasting then feel free to stop and just concentrate on the diet and training. Then when you're ready phase in the fasting after 3 weeks.

The great thing about a fitness model body is they are completely achievable. They aren't some freak of nature with ludicrous conditioning and you won't be starving yourself to the point of being a stick thin waif. You can achieve these physiques if you put the work in.

I'm going to give you a hard-as-nails workout routine to get this physique - the female fitness body.

Here's an interesting fact: you will need to rest sparingly between workouts, and go at a pace right for you. Working out isn't a race to get more muscles or lose more fat than the other person in the gym, but to pace yourself, move progressively forward. Yes it will feel hard, but that means it is working. Luckily every Sunday will give you a well-deserved break and a cheat meal.

If you do want to get into the industry you will need an agent. But to get an agent you need a portfolio and that means a building a fantastic body first! I go into getting an agent in the next chapter.

So let's get started. It's time for you to become an amazing well-toned person with the body of your dreams!

2. How to Get an Agent

If you want to get into commercial modelling then you will need an agent. An agent gets you either direct bookings and/or castings. The higher the job is worth the more likely you will be sent to a casting.

Direct bookings are based on your pictures on an agent's books/website. So getting your pictures done professionally when you're in great shape is key. Going to a casting is a great way to show off your great physique to casting agents. They may not cast you in that job but if you impress - they'll remember you. So obviously you want more direct bookings than castings so we need to look our best.

Preparation:

Firstly you need a set of pictures, which can be relatively normal, they'll want to see what you look like without lots of effects and photoshop. But before you waste time setting up a shoot, you need to look your very best. So schedule in a date for the shoot. For example 5 months from today. Arrange it with a friend, a photographer. Book it in. Mark it in the calendar. That's when you're going to do the shoot.

Now take a picture of yourself in normal lighting conditions. Ask a friend to take a picture with your phone. Take a close up of your face and get someone to take a full length. Now we have a starting point. We want to see the change in you in 5 months. It will be life changing in more ways than one.

Imagine that feeling you will feel when you take a picture of yourself in 5 months? How good is that going to feel when you put the pictures side by side? You will be leaner, sexier and look and feel amazing. And let's not beat around the bush here. That's why we're doing it, not for anyone else, but for us. We want it, we want the change and it starts today.

Getting more pictures

Once you are looking great you don't have to wait around to get an agent. A lot of modelling now is about you being proactive. Here are a list of good websites to join where you can represent yourself:

www.starnow.com

www.castingcallpro.com

www.castingcallpro.co.uk

www.purpleport.com

These websites enable you to join, create a profile and apply for jobs and more importantly get new pictures. Purple port in particular is pretty good for getting Time For Print (TFP) work which means you work for free with a photographer but you'll come away with the images they take. There are many others, so begin looking around on facebook model pages.

A Word of Warning

There are a lot of wannabe photographers, frauds, and generally people who have no idea what they are doing or have ulterior motives - e.g. meeting a hot girl. This should not put you off getting into the industry. But you have to make sure the jobs you are applying for look reputable, the photographers that are offering a shoot should look professional. A professional photographer will have a portfolio of what he has done and you should ask to see that. Even new a photographer should put the effort in to shoot something before working with a model, and have images of landscapes etc. If he hasn't done anything at all then I wouldn't work with him. He needs to learn his craft. If you know someone with a camera then get practicing. If you are approached out of the blue for a shoot - again ask to see what they have done. It's your right to ask. Many times I have been asked to act in shorts, I ask what they have done and don't hear back.

Lastly and obviously don't go to their house for the shoot, you'd meet at the location (not their house!) or studio. I've heard of some horror stories.

Approaching Agents

It is a good idea to get some work from the above websites before approaching agents but not essential. Most applications are done via the agency's website. You'd fill in your bio and include a couple of your pictures. They may ask for 'normal' ones which are selfies or unaltered images. But I'd always include one 'best professional picture' at least. Then move on and approach more. They'll get back to you within around 2 weeks and ask for a meeting.

A word of warning. Some agencies will ask you to pay to join them or worse charge you to update your portfolio. This is a scam. No reputable agency would ask you for money. You are being taken on to make money so they should arrange a shoot if you need more pictures etc. So run the other way if they want to charge you no matter their excuses and reasons.

Social Media

Be proactive here as building a following can have a direct result now to being taken on by some agencies and even being hired through your agent by some clients. Create a fan page on Facebook, an Instagram and Twitter account. Your phone can link all these together so when you post something on Instagram the picture gets posted to all the various accounts.

The # is your special weapon and lots of #model #photographer #modelling #fitness #getfit are all great and the variations.

But first we need the body right?

3. Building The Body You Knew You Had

Let's go into what weeks will be for what workout. As you can see the 10 weeks are varied, with heavy weights weeks separated by heart pumping cardio and then a limbering, calming yoga week. This allows us to really ramp up the muscle toning and leaning and then come down, recuperate during the yoga to go again.

1 - Training Frequency

The training is split into 10 weeks:

Week 1 – High Intensity Interval Training
Week 2 – Weights
Week 3 – High Intensity Interval Training
Week 4 – Yoga
Week 5 – Weights
Week 6 – Cardio
Week 7 – Yoga
Week 8 – Weights
Week 9 – Cardio
Week 10 – Yoga

This is simple, high impact, time friendly and results driven regime.

You should schedule your Training Session to occur in the interval after Breakfast to before Dinner. You should not do a heavy Training Session after the 16-hour fast period (that ends at Breakfast). A walking session, or stretching is fine before Breakfast, but not a high intensity workout.

If you must, then the Training Session can occur an hour or two after Dinner

2 - Body Fat

So this is the number one issue to deal with when beginning a new regime. A low body fat will reveal your body to its best potential. This is also why the weights workouts are supersets combined with cardio. We are ramping up your intensity and effort to burn additional calories.

3 - Nutrition

Nutrition is considered the most important part of building a lean athletic physique. If the nutrition is incorrect then it doesn't matter how impeccable your training routines are, you will not progress. I'm sure you have an idea about nutrition, but I'm here to give your knowledge a little boast. You've heard of high protein, carbohydrates and healthy fats? But what is the most effective foods to eat to get those essential nutrients. So I list each day meal plans which are there for you to follow and create your own by branching off.

We also need to take care to stay hydrated - this cleans our systems, regulates body temperature and keeps the entire body hydrated. So with heavy exercise, 3 litters a day is an ideal figure to aim for.

4. Old Exercises - New Tricks

Let's go into detail about what we'll be doing.

Weights, Cardio and Flexibility Cycle

Weight Weeks

Many women worry that by weight lifting they will become the next Miss Olympia. This isn't the case. You would have to be on a seriously high protein diet and injecting yourself with steroids to come anywhere close. Weight training is becoming the norm for women who want to tone up and get lean. We'll get stronger and build endurance. We'll be training one day on, one off which will consist of cardio. This allows the body to recover as weight training can be draining.

HITT and Cardio Weeks

The second week is all about cardio and toning the overall body. Lots of great fat-burning moves to simple to follow routines. Again I urge you to walk every morning, sometimes we're going to run. Aim to increase walking where possible, it's one of the easiest exercises and safest exercises to do and it all counts. Again Sunday is a rest day and a cheat day, so you can relax and enjoy a cheat meal of your choice.

Yoga Weeks

We'll be focusing on stretching and flexibility. Never stretch further than where your body aches, as this is about relaxing and working out your body. Each day try to extend yourself further and holding your stances longer, but as we won't be building muscles, we won't be taking in as much protein in our diet.

Supersets to Size

If you're unfamiliar with Supersets- they are two exercises working opposite muscles. They are time-efficient method of training that we'll be using during the weight sessions. By doing sets back-to-back, you reduce your total workout time while still doing the same amount of total work.

Super setting is fantastic for pummelling antagonistic muscles - Back/Biceps, Chest/Triceps, Back/Chest and Biceps/Triceps and legs Hams/Glutes. Supersets increase Lactic Acid production, which helps boost Growth Hormone (GH) levels in the body. The body responds to the reduced pH (increased acidity) in the body from the production of Lactic Acid by secreting GH. GH is a powerful fat loss hormone - which is exactly what we want!

Power and Intensity

We will be building more explosive power which will therefore build strength faster. This is done using tempo. By this I mean a 1 second pull/push/ on a given move - POWERFUL and with FORCE - and then under perfect control a 4 second release. The muscles are still working all the way. So we are changing the tempo, the speed of either the concentric (shortening) or eccentric (lengthening) component of the lift. There is no 'resting' at the bottom of any move. As soon as you are as close to the bottom of the move - you POWER back up for the 1 second concentric and again release for 4 second eccentric under your complete control. This should give you a great pump and be a challenge to start with.

Why?

You must have heard of the term TUT - Time Under Tension - there are a number of variations on the term, they all mean the same. You may find that you're actually only working your muscles for 5 minutes in an hour workout! With the 1 second concentric and 4 second eccentric move with no rest we work the muscle much harder for longer.

Many people will struggle with this at first as it's so common to do one arm curl, take a break/release all tension and do another. Even a split second rest is still a release of tension. Not good enough. You need to be working your muscles 100% of the time during a set. THEN you rest between sets.

So let's learn a little more about Intermittent Fasting.

5. Intermittent Fasting Explained

Intermittent Fasting is fairly common within the fitness industry now and many books have been written on its various benefits. I've written a book on the 5:2 method which is about eating normally 5 days a week and eating 500 calories on two separate days. This is the 16:8 method and as I mentioned this squeezes the eating window down to 8 hours and stretches the fasting period to 16 hours.

- Breakfast 12pm
- Lunch 4pm
- Dinner 7pm

16/8 and How it works

You eat within a window of 8 hours, effectively squashing your 3 meals closer together and fast for 16 hours. The fast is where the magic happens. Once you push the body into a fasted state we begin to reap the benefits of Intermittent Fasting:

- Insulin levels: Blood levels of insulin drop significantly, which aids fat burning.

- Human growth hormone: The blood levels of growth hormone may increase as much as 5-fold. Higher levels of this hormone facilitate fat burning and muscle gain, and have many other benefits.

- Cellular repair: The body induces important cellular repair processes, such as removing waste material from cells.

- Gene expression: There are beneficial changes in several genes and molecules related to longevity and protection against disease.

Now combine that with a high energy workout and weights regime and we can create an amazingly leaner sexier body - or put it another way - the best body you always had! The practice of fasting has been around as early as the 1940s and it hasn't been until recently that research has backed up that the true benefits of fasting.

Fasting + Exercise

So this book combines 16/8 fasting and exercise to get to your goals much quicker. We are enhancing and augmenting the fat burning capacity of fasting by incorporating exercise.

So this new health regime is designed to create the best body you already had - but we are going to reveal your amazing lines with hard work and diligence.

We want a visually pleasing physique - strong legs, svelte arms, toned chest, lean back all tapering to and perhaps the most important - a tight taut flat stomach. Sound good? Yep I thought so, let's read on and see how.

To give you a quick overview of how we will achieve this I have broken the training regime down into 4 areas:

Essentially eating in a period of 8 hours and not eating at all for 16 creates a fat-burning environment for your body. So I have created a simple time-table pushing breakfast to 12 midday. I know you're thinking hang on 'I can't go without breakfast!' But trust me, I am doing it right now and you feel more alert and it's really not a problem, but remember all those lovely benefits? No? Scroll up and read them again! Lots of amazing things are happening all pointing to fat loss.

We will be eating from a new meal plan which is designed for you to add and subtract foods. We also want to limit sugar and cut out all refined carbs such as cakes. All these fatty unhealthy foods are doing is adding to the work you need to do to burn them off. However we won't be living like monks and Sunday's are our cheat day, in that we can have a cheat meal and relax the hours of eating.

Instead we will be eating high protein foods and highly nutritious vegetables and fruits.

Liquids

Water is our friend and provides us with many benefits including: can help control calories, helps energize muscles, and helps keep skin looking great. I would try to lower coffee and tea consumption to around 2-3 cups day and get that down to 2 over the course of 2 weeks. I personally love my coffee with milk and 1 sugar and I don't want to cut that out so I have one day.

I would avoid sugary drinks as this will interfere with spiking insulin. We want this effect to be unadulterated. I would stick to water until you reach 12PM.

So without further ado let's begin our journey.

6. Week 1 Workout - HIIT

Monday – HIIT weeks begins

So here we are at the start of a amazing journey to slim down, look great and more importantly feel great. We want to rev up your metabolism so we will be doing cardio in the morning before breakfast.

We will be making use of a pedometer that almost every smart phone has. I want you to be doing 6000 steps a day this week on top of your cardio. That roughly equates to 1 hour of walking. Just work this into getting to and from work and a walk on your lunch break and it'll be done without even trying.

To maximize the benefits of a cardio workout, you have to elevate your heart rate and keep it elevated for at least 20 consecutive minutes. You will want to monitor your heart rate during the workouts. This will improve your heart and lung function.

IF YOU ARE OVER 40 YEARS OLD, OR HAVE A HISTORY OF HEART DISEASE, THEN YOU SHOULD BE MEDICALLY CLEARED BY YOUR PHYSICIAN BEFORE STARTING ANY CARDIO EXERCISE PROGRAM.

The formula for your target heart rate is based on your theoretical maximum heart rate. Subtract your age from 220. This is your maximum heart rate. Your target rate is 60-80% of the maximum.

For example- if you are 20, your maximum heart rate is 200. The target rate is 120-160. So you need to exercise at a level that raises your heart rate to this range and keeps it there for at least 20 minutes.

Let's ramp up the fat burning and get down to it!

Workout – Fasted Cardio:

Firstly you will need:

A wall clock or a large stop watch. This is so you don't keep stopping to check your phone. Once you start you don't want to stop until you've reached the end.

So we will do 4 exercises x 4 for a total 16 minutes – we will work hard for 30 seconds of the exercise giving everything we have and rest for 30 seconds. Then we move onto the next exercise – do 30 seconds as hard as we can and rest and so on until we complete the workout. This will feel very tough to start with but trust me you'll love the feeling afterwards.

Round 1

- **Running on the spot – keeping the knees as high as you can all the way**
- Rest 30 seconds
- **Burpees**
- Rest 30 seconds
- **Press-ups**
- Rest 30 seconds
- **Jumping Jacks**

- Rest 30 seconds - **Get ready and here we go!**

Round 2

- **Running on the spot – keeping the knees as high as you can all the way**
- Rest 30 seconds
- **Burpees**
- Rest 30 seconds
- **Press-ups**
- Rest 30 seconds
- **Jumping Jacks**
- Rest 30 seconds - **Get ready and here we go!**

Round 3

- **Running on the spot – keeping the knees as high as you can all the way**
- Rest 30 seconds
- **Burpees**
- Rest 30 seconds
- **Press-ups**
- Rest 30 seconds
- **Jumping Jacks**

- Rest 30 seconds - **Get ready and here we go!**

Round 4

- **Running on the spot – keeping the knees as high as you can all the way**
- Rest 30 seconds
- **Burpees**
- Rest 30 seconds
- **Press-ups**
- Rest 30 seconds
- **Jumping Jacks**

And Rest – well done – go grab a drink!

Nutrition

Upon Waking:

Have a long glass of warm water with lemon - either fresh lemon or pure lemon dripped in.

Then do your Fasted Cardio workout above – no excuses, it's only 20 minutes including warm ups. Drink plenty of water after your workout.

12 P.M - Breakfast - Meal One

- 1 x multivitamin
- 2 Whole Eggs Scrambled
- Mixed with Green beans cut up

NUTRITION FACTS

Calories: 409   Fat: 17.6 g   Carbs: 20.6 g   Protein: 16.3 g

4 P.M - Lunch - Meal Two

- 1 Can of Tuna Steak
- Red bell peppers, and low fat Coleslaw

NUTRITION FACTS

Calories: 386   Fat: 17g   Carbs: 17g   Protein: 27g

7 P.M - Dinner - Meal Three

- Chicken Breast - With parsley, and bell peppers sliced up
- Peas and Carrots

NUTRITION FACTS

Calories: 318   Fat: 15g   Carbs: 15g   Protein: 24g

The Total Protein intake is 67.3 grams of protein. I would have 1 scoop of protein - 25grams - after your workout making a grand total of 92.3.

Notice how the carbs are minimal - except after your training. You can have carbs then, then stick with veg and fruit.

Tuesday - Cardio

Before Breakfast:

Very simple, do your 5 minute warm up and then go for an early 30 minute run - outside or use the running machine in a gym.

Be sure to warm down.

Plus, remember lots of walking today - as much as you can.

Nutrition

Upon Waking:

Have a long glass of warm water with lemon - either fresh lemon or pure lemon dripped in before your workout.

12 P.M - Breakfast - Meal One

- 1 x multivitamin
- 1 x Whey Protein shake - with peanut butter and a banana
- 1 30gram x Bowl of Granola

NUTRITION FACTS

Calories: 561   Fat: 30.4 g   Carbs: 26.2 g   Protein: 28 g

4 P.M - Lunch - Meal Two

- 1 x Medium sized Tuna Steak
- 1 x Cup Vegetables/salad

NUTRITION FACTS

Calories: 471   Fat: 33.2 g   Carbs: 17 g   Protein: 27 g

7 PM - Dinner - Meal Three

- Tuna Steak
- Rocket and sliced Red Peppers
- Medium Sweet Potato

NUTRITION FACTS

Calories: 456   Fat: 17g Carbs: 29g   Protein: 28g

The Total Protein intake is 83 grams of protein. I would have 1 scoops of protein plus after your workout making a grand total of 108.

Wednesday - Cardio

Workout – Fasted Cardio:

So we will do 4 exercises x 4 for a total 16 minutes – we will work hard for 30 seconds of the exercise giving everything we have and rest for 30 seconds. Then we move onto the next exercise – do 30 seconds as hard as we can and rest and so on until we complete the workout. This will feel very tough to start with but trust me you'll love the feeling afterwards.

Round 1

- **Running on the spot – while punching**
- Rest 30 seconds
- **Burpees**
- Rest 30 seconds
- **Star Jumps**
- Rest 30 seconds
- **Mountain Climbers**

- Rest 30 seconds - **Get ready and here we go!**

Round 2

- **Running on the spot – while punching**
- Rest 30 seconds
- **Burpees**
- Rest 30 seconds
- **Star Jumps**
- Rest 30 seconds
- **Mountain Climbers**

- Rest 30 seconds - **Get ready and here we go!**

Round 3

- **Running on the spot – while punching**
- Rest 30 seconds
- **Burpees**
- Rest 30 seconds
- **Star Jumps**
- Rest 30 seconds
- **Mountain Climbers**

- Rest 30 seconds - **Get ready and here we go!**

Round 4

- **Running on the spot – while punching**
- Rest 30 seconds
- **Burpees**
- Rest 30 seconds
- **Star Jumps**
- Rest 30 seconds
- **Mountain Climbers**

And you've finished – go get a drink!

Nutrition

<u>Upon Waking:</u>

Have 2 long glasses of warm water with lemon - either fresh lemon or pure lemon dripped in. Now do your fasted cardio as above and drink plenty afterwards.

12 P.M - Breakfast - Meal One

- 1 x multivitamin
- 2 boiled eggs
- Porridge Oats 30gram serving with 1 tbsp. honey

NUTRITION FACTS

Calories: 409   Fat: 17.6 g   Carbs: 35.6 g   Protein: 20.3 g

4 P.M - Lunch - Meal Two

- Full-Fat Cottage Cheese
- 1 cup Cashews
- 1 Pear
- 1 Banana

NUTRITION FACTS

Calories: 566   Fat: 17 g Carb: 59 g   Protein: 28 g

7 P.M - Dinner - Meal Three

- Pork Chops 5 ounces- with cooked apple - cooked together
- Vegetables 1 cup

NUTRITION FACTS

Calories: 380   Fat: 18.2 g   Carbs: 25 g   Protein: 28 g

The Total Protein intake is 76.3 grams of protein. I would have 1 scoop of protein after your workout making a grand total of 101.3.

Thursday - Cardio

Before Breakfast:

Very simple, do my Warm Up routine and then go for an early 25 minutes of spinning or a bike ride - outside or use the running machine in a gym.

Or just stick to the pavement and do a 30 minute run.

Be sure to warm down.

Nutrition

Upon Waking:

Have a long glass of warm water with lemon - either fresh lemon or pure lemon dripped in. Do your exercise as above and remember to drink at least 2 glasses of water afterwards.

12 P.M - Breakfast - Meal One

- 1 x multivitamin
- 1 x Whey Protein shake - with peanut butter and a banana
- 1 30gram x Bowl of Granola

NUTRITION FACTS

Calories: 561   Fat: 30.4 g   Carbs: 26.2 g   Protein: 28 g

4 P.M Lunch - Meal Two

- 1 x can of Tuna Steak
- Rocket and Beetroot

NUTRITION FACTS

Calories: 471   Fat: 33.2 g   Carbs: 17 g   Protein: 27 g

7 P.M Dinner - Meal Three

- Chicken Breast - With parsley, and bell peppers sliced up
- Steamed Broccoli

NUTRITION FACTS

Calories: 318   Fat: 15g   Carbs: 15g   Protein: 24g

The Total Protein intake is 79 grams of protein. I would have 1 scoops of protein plus after your workout making a grand total of 104.

Friday - Cardio

Workout – Fasted Cardio:

So we will do 4 exercises x 4 for a total 16 minutes – we will work hard for 30 seconds of the exercise giving everything we have and rest for 30 seconds. Then we move onto the next exercise – do 30 seconds as hard as we can and rest and so on until we complete the workout. This will feel very tough to start with but trust me you'll love the feeling afterwards.

Round 1

- **Skip Rope – use an imaginary rope to skip**
- Rest 30 seconds
- **Burpees**
- Rest 30 seconds
- **Press-ups**
- Rest 30 seconds
- **Squats with a Shoulder Press at the top**

- Rest 30 seconds - **Get ready and here we go!**

Round 2

- **Skip Rope – use an imaginary rope to skip**
- Rest 30 seconds
- **Burpees**
- Rest 30 seconds
- **Press-ups**
- Rest 30 seconds
- **Squats with a Shoulder Press at the top**

- Rest 30 seconds - **Get ready and here we go!**

Round 3

- **Skip Rope – use an imaginary rope to skip**
- Rest 30 seconds
- **Burpees**
- Rest 30 seconds
- **Press-ups**
- Rest 30 seconds
- **Squats with a Shoulder Press at the top**

- Rest 30 seconds - **Get ready and here we go!**

Round 4

- **Skip Rope – use an imaginary rope to skip**
- Rest 30 seconds
- **Burpees**
- Rest 30 seconds
- **Press-ups**
- Rest 30 seconds
- **Squats with a Shoulder Press at the top**

And Rest – well done – go grab a drink!

Nutrition

Upon Waking:

Have 2 glasses of warm water with lemon - either fresh lemon or pure lemon dripped in. Do your fasted cardio and then drink plenty.

12 P.M - Breakfast - Meal One

- 1 x multivitamin
- 2 Whole Eggs Scrambled
- Mixed with Green beans cut up

NUTRITION FACTS

Calories: 409   Fat: 17.6 g   Carbs: 20.6 g   Protein: 16.3 g

4 P.M Lunch - Meal Two

- 1 x Medium sized Tuna Steak
- 1 x Cup Vegetables/salad
- 1 Medium sized Baked Potato

NUTRITION FACTS

Calories: 571   Fat: 33.2 g   Carbs: 80 g   Protein: 33 g

7 P.M - Dinner - Meal Three

- Chicken Breast - With parsley, and bell peppers sliced up
- Sprouts - cooked and mashed - add pepper and soft cheese - mash up

NUTRITION FACTS

Calories: 418   Fat: 15g   Carbs: 28g   Protein: 29g

The Total Protein intake is 78.3 grams of protein. I would have 1 scoop of protein - 25grams - after your workout making a grand total of 103.3.

Saturday - Cardio

Before Breakfast

1 hour of swimming - or 1 x 45 minute insanity workout – or do Mondays HIIT.

In terms of swimming I want to mix it up, this is also very low impact, your muscles could probably do with something relaxing. Try to put in lengths and keep moving.

Again warming up and cooling down is very important.

Nutrition

Upon Waking:

Have a long glass of warm water with lemon - either fresh lemon or pure lemon dripped in.

12 P.M - Breakfast - Meal One

- 1 x multivitamin
- 2 boiled eggs
- Porridge Oats 30gram serving with 1 tbsp. honey

NUTRITION FACTS

Calories: 409   Fat: 17.6 g   Carbs: 35.6 g   Protein: 20.3 g

4 P.M - Lunch - Meal Two

- Full-Fat Cottage Cheese
- 1 cups Cashews
- 1 Apple

NUTRITION FACTS

Calories: 356   Fat: 17 g Carb: 9 g   Protein: 26 g

7 P.M - Dinner - Meal Three

- Pork Chops 5 ounces- with cooked apple - cooked together
- Vegetables 1 cup

NUTRITION FACTS

Calories: 380   Fat: 18.2 g   Carbs: 25 g   Protein: 28 g

The Total Protein intake is 74.3 grams of protein. I would have 1 scoop of protein after your workout making a grand total of 99.3.

7. Week 2 Weights Workout

Week two begins and we will start our weights routine to tone muscle, burn fat and get stronger. We will train one day on weights and the next day off. This allows the muscles and systems of the body to recover and grow.

When to train?

Personally I have got into a routine of training early in the morning. This initially seems awful however wait until you do it. You will feel amazing afterwards, and especially when you feel you have earnt a hearty breakfast. The rest of the day is spent burning fat because you've kick started your body. Plus any other exercise you do such as walking etc is a bonus, you're done and dusted. If you can't then train before dinner, so dinner becomes your post workout meal.

So let's start with one of the biggest groups – legs. Fantastic for building overall strength and conditioning - let's go.

Monday - Legs and Calves

Walk: 25-minute walk early to work, or before work round the block - it's leg day and so don't need to do anything too hard.

Round 1

I would certainly do this work out after work, amongst your feeding time so you have energy to train and can replace energy. Warm up thoroughly. Increase the weight little by little with each set.

Exercise	Sets/Reps
BARBELL SQUAT	2 warm up light sets, 3 sets of 12, 10, 8 reps
STANDING LEG CURL	3 sets of 15, 12, 10 reps
SMITH MACHINE LEG PRESS	3 sets of 8 reps

Do the Barbell Squat separately, and Superset the Standing Leg Curl and Leg Press

Round 2

Increase the weight little by little with each set.

Exercise	Sets/Reps
DEADLIFT	3 sets of 12, 10, 8 reps
LEG EXTENSIONS	3 sets of 15, 12, 10 reps
LEG CURLS	3 sets of 10 reps

Do the Deadlift separately, and Superset the Leg Extensions and Leg Curls

Round 3

Increase the weight little by little with each set.

Exercise	Sets/Reps
STANDING CALF RAISES	3 sets of 12, 10, 8 reps
Superset	
SEATED CALF RAISE	3 sets of 12-15 reps

Nutrition

Upon Waking:

Have a long glass of warm water with lemon - either fresh lemon or pure lemon dripped in.

12 P.M - Breakfast - Meal One

- 1 x multivitamin
- 2 Whole Eggs Scrambled
- Mixed with Green beans cut up

NUTRITION FACTS

Calories: 409   Fat: 17.6 g   Carbs: 20.6 g   Protein: 16.3 g

4 P.M - Lunch - Meal Two

- Chicken Breast - With parsley, and bell peppers sliced up
- Vegetables - 1-2 cups

NUTRITION FACTS

Calories: 318   Fat: 15g   Carbs: 15g   Protein: 24g

7 PM - Dinner - Meal Three

- Tuna Steak
- Rocket and sliced Red Peppers
- Medium Sweet Potato

NUTRITION FACTS

Calories: 456   Fat: 17g   Carbs: 29g   Protein: 28g

The Total Protein intake is 68.3 grams of protein. I would have 1 scoop of protein - 25grams - after your workout making a grand total of 93.3.

Notice how the carbs are minimal - except after your training. You can have carbs then, then stick with veg and fruit.

Tuesday - Abs/Cardio + Nutrition

Upon Waking:

Have a long glass of warm water with lemon - either fresh lemon or pure lemon dripped in.

Before Breakfast: These can be done later in the day

3 sets- 20 Crunches each set

3 sets- 25 Standing Twists each direction

3 sets- 20 Side-Lying Leg Lifts each direction

Run: Again, do this later in the day, at least after the first meal.

25-minute run (remember to warm up and down)
Try to walk as much as possible, later on to from work or to a further station etc.

12 P.M - Breakfast - Meal One

- 1 x multivitamin
- 1 x Whey Protein shake - with peanut butter and a banana
- 1 30gram x Bowl of Granola

NUTRITION FACTS

Calories: 561   Fat: 30.4 g   Carbs: 26.2 g   Protein: 28 g

4 P.M - Lunch - Meal Two

- 1 x Medium sized Tuna Steak
- 1 x Cup Vegetables/salad

NUTRITION FACTS

Calories: 471   Fat: 33.2 g   Carbs: 17 g   Protein: 27

7 P.M - Dinner - Meal Three

- 2 Large Eggs Omelette with chopped green beans
- 2 Rice Cakes
- 1 x Peach

NUTRITION FACTS

Calories: 349   Fat: 14 g Carb: 25 g   Protein: 16 g

The Total Protein intake is 71 grams of protein. I would have 1 scoops of protein plus after your workout making a grand total of 96.

Wednesday - Chest and Triceps

Walk: 30 Minute brisk walk before breakfast - again breakfast is ideal.

Weights- Mid-afternoon is best.

Round 1

Increase the weight little by little with each set. 45 second break between sets.

Exercise	Sets/Reps
BARBELL BENCH PRESS - MEDIUM GRIP	1-2 sets of 15 reps (warm-up); 3 sets of 12, 10, 8 reps
Superset	
LYING TRICEPS PRESS	3 sets of 15, 12, 10 reps

Superset the Bench Press and Triceps Press

Round 2

Increase the weight little by little with each set.

Exercise	Sets/Reps
BARBELL INCLINE BENCH PRESS	3 sets of 12, 10, 8 reps
Superset	
TRICEPS PUSHDOWN	3 sets of 15, 12, 10 reps

Superset the Incline Bench Press and Triceps Pushdown

Round 3

Increase the weight little by little with each set.

Exercise	Sets/Reps
DUMBBELL FLYS	3 sets of 12, 10, 8 reps
Superset	
CABLE ROPE OVERHEAD TRICEPS EXTENSION	3 sets of 15, 12, 8 reps

Superset the Flies and Triceps Overhead Pulls

You can add a set of Push Ups at the end

Nutrition

Upon Waking:

Have a long glass of warm water with lemon - either fresh lemon or pure lemon dripped in.

12 P.M - Breakfast - Meal One

- 1 x multivitamin
- 2 boiled eggs
- Porridge Oats 30gram serving with 1 tbsp. honey

NUTRITION FACTS

Calories: 409   Fat: 17.6 g   Carbs: 35.6 g   Protein: 20.3 g

4 P.M - Lunch - Meal Two

- Pork Chops 5 ounces- with cooked apple - cooked together
- Vegetables 1 cup

NUTRITION FACTS

Calories: 380   Fat: 18.2 g   Carbs: 25 g   Protein: 28 g

7 P.M - Dinner - Meal Three

- Full-Fat Cottage Cheese
- 1 cup Cashews
- 1 Apple
- 1 Banana

NUTRITION FACTS

Calories: 556   Fat: 17 g Carb: 59 g   Protein: 28 g

The Total Protein intake is 76.3 grams of protein. I would have 1 scoop of protein after your workout making a grand total of 101.3.

Thursday - Abs/Cardio + Nutrition

Upon Waking:

Have a long glass of warm water with lemon - either fresh lemon or pure lemon dripped in.

Run: 30-minute run. I'd like you to get in a good 30-minute walk at the end of the day.

After work:

3 sets of 30 Twists each side

3 set of Side Bends each side- if too easy, add a 5-10 pound dumbbell

4 sets of Hold plank – 30 seconds each

12 P.M - Breakfast - Meal One

- 1 x multivitamin
- 2 Whole Eggs Scrambled
- Mixed with Green beans cut up

NUTRITION FACTS

Calories: 409   Fat: 17.6 g   Carbs: 20.6 g   Protein: 16.3 g

4 P.M - Lunch - Meal Two

- Chicken Breast - With parsley, and bell peppers sliced up
- Steamed Broccoli

NUTRITION FACTS

Calories: 318   Fat: 15g   Carbs: 15g   Protein: 24g

7 PM - Dinner - Meal Three

- Tuna Steak
- Cucumber, tomatoes, Wild Rocket and Celery chunks

NUTRITION FACTS

Calories: 376   Fat: 17g   Carbs: 9g   Protein: 27g

The Total Protein intake is 67.3 grams of protein. I would have 1 scoop of protein - 25grams - after your workout making a grand total of 92.3.

Notice how the carbs are minimal - except after your training. You can have carbs then, then stick with veg and fruit.

Friday - Back and Biceps

Walk: 30 Minutes of cardio before breakfast. We want to burn fat before anything else and get the body prepared for the day.

Round 1

Increase the weight little by little with each set. 45 second between sets.

Exercise	Sets/Reps
CHIN-UP	1-2 sets of 15 reps (warm-up); 3 sets of 12, 10, 8 reps
Superset	
BARBELL CURL	3 sets of 10-12 reps

If you cannot do many (or any) Chin-Ups, then stand on a stool to support some of your body weight. Hang down, and do the Chin-Up, pulling as hard as you can to pull up to the bar, and supporting as little of your weight on one foot.

Superset the Chin-Ups with the Barbell Curls- do one Chin-Up set, then a Barbell set, then repeat until finished.

Round 2

Increase the weight little by little with each set.

Exercise	Sets/Reps
WIDE-GRIP REAR PULL-UP	3 sets of 15, 12, 10 reps
Superset	
DUMBBELL ALTERNATE BICEP CURL	3 sets of 10-12 reps

Same as above if you cannot do many (or any) Pull-Ups.

Superset the Pull-Up sets with the Dumbbell Biceps Curls.

Round 3

Increase the weight little by little with each set.

Exercise	Sets/Reps
T-BAR ROW	3 sets of 15, 12, 8 reps
Superset	
INCLINE DUMBBELL REVERSE CURL	3 sets of 10-12 rep

Superset the Rows with the Dumbbell Reverse Curls. Reverse Curl means that your hands are facing away as you flex your elbow.

Nutrition

Upon Waking:

Have a long glass of warm water with lemon - either fresh lemon or pure lemon dripped in.

12 P.M - Breakfast - Meal One

- 1 x multivitamin
- 1 x Whey Protein shake - with peanut butter and a banana
- 1 30gram x Bowl of Granola

NUTRITION FACTS

Calories: 561   Fat: 30.4 g   Carbs: 26.2 g   Protein: 28 g

4 P.M - Lunch - Meal Two

- Greek Yogurt - High Protein
- 1 x Sliced Peach
- 2 cups Cashews

NUTRITION FACTS

Calories: 752   Fat: 34 g Carb: 18 g   Protein: 52 g

7 P.M - Dinner - Meal Three

- 1 x Medium sized Tuna Steak
- 1 x Cup Vegetables/salad
- 1 Medium sized Baked Potato

NUTRITION FACTS

Calories: 571   Fat: 33.2 g   Carbs: 80 g   Protein: 33 g

I've given you a huge carb dinner here after the leg workout and this will replenish your energy. Add a dab of butter too. The Total Protein intake is 113 grams of protein. I would have 1 scoops of protein plus after your workout making a grand total of 138.

Saturday - Abs/Cardio + Nutrition

Upon Waking:

Have a long glass of warm water with lemon - either fresh lemon or pure lemon dripped in.

Before Breakfast: - Ab Blast

20 x Crunches

25 x Twists

15 x sit-ups

20 x Crunches

25 x Twists

15 x sit-ups

20 x Crunches

25 x Twists

15 x sit-ups

Run: 30 minute run - during the morning.

12 P.M - Breakfast - Meal One

- 1 x multivitamin
- 1 Whole Egg
- 1 piece of salmon
- Oats 1/4 cup with 1 tbsp. honey

NUTRITION FACTS

Calories: 561   Fat: 30.4 g   Carbs: 20.2 g   Protein: 26.1 g

4 P.M - Lunch - Meal Two

- High Protein Frozen Yogurt
- Cashews 2 ounces
- 1 Apple

NUTRITION FACTS

Calories: 356   Fat: 17 g Carb: 9 g   Protein: 26 g

7 P.M - Dinner - Meal Four

- Pork Chops 5 ounces- with cooked apple - cooked together
- Vegetables 1 cup

NUTRITION FACTS

Calories: 380   Fat: 18.2 g   Carbs: 25 g   Protein: 28 g

The Total Protein intake is 80.1 grams of protein. I would have 1 scoop of protein after your workout making a grand total of 105.1.

Sunday - Rest

So we've made it to our rest day - well done for an epic week 1 of workouts! You should be feeling good, a little achy maybe, but you got through it. Did you miss any workouts? If so, it doesn't matter, let's go one better this coming week. It's about progression.

So today is all about chilling, eating well, having your cheat meal - which is anything of your choice. Also it's Sunday so you don't need to follow the strict eating times if you want a break. Not that it should ever feel a chore, but having breakfast at the old breakfast time never hurt anyone on a Sunday.

Upon Waking:

Have a long glass of warm water with lemon - either fresh lemon or pure lemon dripped in.

Breakfast - Meal One

- 1 x multivitamin
- 3 x scrambled eggs - with spinach
- 1 30gram x Bowl of Granola

NUTRITION FACTS

Calories: 561   Fat: 30.4 g   Carbs: 26.2 g   Protein: 26 g

Lunch - Meal Two

CHEAT MEAL - whatever you fancy!

7 P.M - Dinner - Meal Three

- 1 Cup x Full-Fat Cottage Cheese
- 1 x blob of peanut butter mixed in

NUTRITION FACTS

Calories: 371   Fat: 27 g Carb: 9 g   Protein: 24 g

For future cheat meals, I'm not going into your exact macros here. Eat well and enjoy yourself until tomorrow.

8. Week 3 Workout - HIIT

Monday – HIIT weeks begins

So here we are at the start of week 3 of our new journey to slim down, and look great. We want to rev up your metabolism this week so we will be doing cardio in the morning before breakfast.

We will making use of a pedometer that almost every smart phone has. I want you to be doing 6000 steps a day this week on top of your cardio. That roughly equates to 1 hour of walking. Just work this into getting to and from work and a walk on your lunch break and it'll be done without even trying.

You will need:

Again you'll need a stopwatch on your phone, or a clock to see. A kitchen type clock is great as you won't need to keep learning forward to see it.

Let's ramp up the fat burning and get down to it!

Workout – Fasted Cardio:

So we will do 4 exercises x 4 for a total 16 minutes – we will work hard for 30 seconds of the exercise giving everything we have and rest for 30 seconds. Then we move onto the next exercise – do 30 seconds as hard as we can and rest and so on until we complete the workout.

Round 1

- **Mountain climbers**
- Rest 30 seconds
- **Burpees**
- Rest 30 seconds
- **Press-ups**
- Rest 30 seconds
- **High Knees on the spot – fast as you can**

- Rest 30 seconds - **Get ready and here we go!**

Round 2

- **Mountain Climbers**
- Rest 30 seconds
- **Burpees**
- Rest 30 seconds
- **Press-ups**
- Rest 30 seconds
- **High Knees**

- Rest 30 seconds - **Get ready and here we go!**

Round 3

- **Mountain Climbers**
- Rest 30 seconds
- **Burpees**
- Rest 30 seconds
- **Press-ups**
- Rest 30 seconds
- **High Knees**

- Rest 30 seconds - **Get ready and here we go!**

Round 4

- **Mountain climbers**
- Rest 30 seconds
- **Burpees**
- Rest 30 seconds
- **Press-ups**
- Rest 30 seconds
- **High Knees**

And Rest – well done – go grab a drink!

Nutrition

Upon Waking:

Have a long glass of warm water with lemon - either fresh lemon or pure lemon dripped in.

Then do your Fasted Cardio workout above – no excuses, it's only 20 minutes including warm ups. Drink plenty of water after your workout.

12 P.M - Breakfast - Meal One

- 1 x multivitamin
- 2 Whole Eggs Scrambled
- Mixed with Green beans cut up

NUTRITION FACTS

Calories: 409   Fat: 17.6 g   Carbs: 20.6 g   Protein: 16.3 g

4 P.M - Lunch - Meal Two

- 1 Can of Tuna Steak
- Red bell peppers, and low fat Coleslaw

NUTRITION FACTS

Calories: 386   Fat: 17g   Carbs: 17g   Protein: 27g

7 P.M - Dinner - Meal Three

- Chicken Breast - With parsley, and bell peppers sliced up
- Peas and Carrots

NUTRITION FACTS

Calories: 318   Fat: 15g   Carbs: 15g   Protein: 24g

The Total Protein intake is 67.3 grams of protein. I would have 1 scoop of protein - 25grams - after your workout making a grand total of 92.3.

Notice how the carbs are minimal - except after your training. You can have carbs then, then stick with veg and fruit.

Tuesday - Cardio

Before Breakfast:

Very simple, do your 5 minute warm up and then go for an early 30 minute run - outside or use the running machine in a gym.

Be sure to warm down.

Plus, remember lots of walking today - as much as you can.

Nutrition

Upon Waking:

Have a long glass of warm water with lemon - either fresh lemon or pure lemon dripped in before your workout.

12 P.M - Breakfast - Meal One

- 1 x multivitamin
- 1 x Whey Protein shake - with peanut butter and a banana
- 1 30gram x Bowl of Granola

NUTRITION FACTS

Calories: 561   Fat: 30.4 g   Carbs: 26.2 g   Protein: 28 g

4 P.M - Lunch - Meal Two

- 1 x Medium sized Tuna Steak
- 1 x Cup Vegetables/salad

NUTRITION FACTS

Calories: 471   Fat: 33.2 g   Carbs: 17 g   Protein: 27 g

7 PM - Dinner - Meal Three

- Tuna Steak
- Rocket and sliced Red Peppers
- Medium Sweet Potato

NUTRITION FACTS

Calories: 456   Fat: 17g   Carbs: 29g   Protein: 28g

The Total Protein intake is 83 grams of protein. I would have 1 scoops of protein plus after your workout making a grand total of 108.

Wednesday - Cardio

Workout – Fasted Cardio:

So we will do 4 exercises x 4 for a total 16 minutes – we will work hard for 30 seconds of the exercise giving everything we have and rest for 30 seconds. Then we move onto the next exercise – do 30 seconds as hard as we can and rest and so on until we complete the workout. This will feel very tough to start with but trust me you'll love the feeling afterwards.

Round 1

- **Running on the spot – while punching**
- Rest 30 seconds
- **Burpees**
- Rest 30 seconds
- **Squat and jump up Shooting for the hoop**
- Rest 30 seconds
- **Mountain Climbers**

- Rest 30 seconds - **Get ready and here we go!**

Round 2

- **Running on the spot – while punching**
- Rest 30 seconds
- **Burpees**
- Rest 30 seconds
- **Squat and jump up Shooting for the hoop**
- Rest 30 seconds
- **Mountain Climbers**

- Rest 30 seconds - **Get ready and here we go!**

Round 3

- **Running on the spot – while punching**
- Rest 30 seconds
- **Burpees**
- Rest 30 seconds
- **Squat and jump up Shooting for the hoop**
- Rest 30 seconds
- **Mountain Climbers**

- Rest 30 seconds - **Get ready and here we go!**

Round 4

- **Running on the spot – while punching**
- Rest 30 seconds
- **Burpees**
- Rest 30 seconds
- **Squat and jump up Shooting for the hoop**
- Rest 30 seconds
- **Mountain Climbers**

And you've finished – go get a drink!

Nutrition

<u>Upon Waking:</u>

Have 2 long glasses of warm water with lemon - either fresh lemon or pure lemon dripped in. Now do your fasted cardio as above and drink plenty afterwards.

12 P.M - Breakfast - Meal One

- 1 x multivitamin
- 2 boiled eggs
- Porridge Oats 30gram serving with 1 tbsp. honey

NUTRITION FACTS

Calories: 409   Fat: 17.6 g   Carbs: 35.6 g   Protein: 20.3 g

4 P.M - Lunch - Meal Two

- Full-Fat Cottage Cheese
- 1 cup Cashews
- 1 Pear
- 1 Banana

NUTRITION FACTS

Calories: 566   Fat: 17 g Carb: 59 g   Protein: 28 g

7 P.M - Dinner - Meal Three

- Pork Chops 5 ounces- with cooked apple - cooked together
- Vegetables 1 cup

NUTRITION FACTS

Calories: 380   Fat: 18.2 g   Carbs: 25 g   Protein: 28 g

The Total Protein intake is 76.3 grams of protein. I would have 1 scoop of protein after your workout making a grand total of 101.3.

Thursday - Cardio

Before Breakfast:

Very simple, do my Warm Up routine and then go for an early 25 minutes of spinning or a bike ride - outside or use the running machine in a gym.

Or just stick to the pavement and do a 30 minute run.

Be sure to warm down.

Nutrition

Upon Waking:

Have a long glass of warm water with lemon - either fresh lemon or pure lemon dripped in. Do your exercise as above and remember to drink at least 2 glasses of water afterwards.

12 P.M - Breakfast - Meal One

- 1 x multivitamin
- 1 x Whey Protein shake - with peanut butter and a banana
- 1 30gram x Bowl of Granola

NUTRITION FACTS

Calories: 561   Fat: 30.4 g   Carbs: 26.2 g   Protein: 28 g

4 P.M Lunch - Meal Two

- 1 x can of Tuna Steak
- Rocket and Beetroot

NUTRITION FACTS

Calories: 471   Fat: 33.2 g   Carbs: 17 g   Protein: 27 g

7 P.M Dinner - Meal Three

- Chicken Breast - With parsley, and bell peppers sliced up
- Steamed Broccoli

NUTRITION FACTS

Calories: 318   Fat: 15g   Carbs: 15g   Protein: 24g

The Total Protein intake is 79 grams of protein. I would have 1 scoops of protein plus after your workout making a grand total of 104.

Friday - Cardio

Workout – Fasted Cardio:

So we will do 4 exercises x 4 for a total 16 minutes – we will work hard for 30 seconds of the exercise giving everything we have and rest for 30 seconds. Then we move onto the next exercise – do 30 seconds as hard as we can and rest and so on until we complete the workout. This will feel very tough to start with but trust me you'll love the feeling afterwards.

Round 1

- **Skip Rope – use an imaginary rope to skip**
- Rest 30 seconds
- **Burpees**
- Rest 30 seconds
- **Press-ups**
- Rest 30 seconds
- **Squats with a Shoulder Press at the top**

- Rest 30 seconds - **Get ready and here we go!**

Round 2

- **Skip Rope – use an imaginary rope to skip**
- Rest 30 seconds
- **Burpees**
- Rest 30 seconds
- **Press-ups**
- Rest 30 seconds
- **Squats with a Shoulder Press at the top**

- Rest 30 seconds - **Get ready and here we go!**

Round 3

- **Skip Rope – use an imaginary rope to skip**
- Rest 30 seconds
- **Burpees**
- Rest 30 seconds
- **Press-ups**
- Rest 30 seconds
- **Squats with a Shoulder Press at the top**

- Rest 30 seconds - **Get ready and here we go!**

Round 4

- **Skip Rope – use an imaginary rope to skip**
- Rest 30 seconds
- **Burpees**
- Rest 30 seconds
- **Press-ups**
- Rest 30 seconds
- **Squats with a Shoulder Press at the top**

And Rest – well done – go grab a drink!

Nutrition

Upon Waking:

Have 2 glasses of warm water with lemon - either fresh lemon or pure lemon dripped in. Do your fasted cardio and then drink plenty.

12 P.M - Breakfast - Meal One

- 1 x multivitamin
- 2 Whole Eggs Scrambled
- Mixed with Green beans cut up

NUTRITION FACTS

Calories: 409   Fat: 17.6 g   Carbs: 20.6 g   Protein: 16.3 g

4 P.M Lunch - Meal Two

- 1 x Medium sized Tuna Steak
- 1 x Cup Vegetables/salad
- 1 Medium sized Baked Potato

NUTRITION FACTS

Calories: 571   Fat: 33.2 g   Carbs: 80 g   Protein: 33 g

7 P.M - Dinner - Meal Three

- Chicken Breast - With parsley, and bell peppers sliced up
- Sprouts - cooked and mashed - add pepper and soft cheese - mash up

NUTRITION FACTS

Calories: 418   Fat: 15g   Carbs: 28g   Protein: 29g

The Total Protein intake is 78.3 grams of protein. I would have 1 scoop of protein - 25grams - after your workout making a grand total of 103.3.

Saturday - Cardio

Before Breakfast

1 hour of swimming - or 1 x 45 minute insanity workout – or do Mondays HIIT.

In terms of swimming I want to mix it up, this is also very low impact, your muscles could probably do with something relaxing. Try to put in lengths and keep moving.

Again warming up and cooling down is very important.

Nutrition

Upon Waking:

Have a long glass of warm water with lemon - either fresh lemon or pure lemon dripped in.

12 P.M - Breakfast - Meal One

- 1 x multivitamin
- 2 boiled eggs
- Porridge Oats 30gram serving with 1 tbsp. honey

NUTRITION FACTS

Calories: 409   Fat: 17.6 g   Carbs: 35.6 g   Protein: 20.3 g

4 P.M - Lunch - Meal Two

- Full-Fat Cottage Cheese
- 1 cups Cashews
- 1 Apple

NUTRITION FACTS

Calories: 356   Fat: 17 g Carb: 9 g   Protein: 26 g

7 P.M - Dinner - Meal Three

- Pork Chops 5 ounces- with cooked apple - cooked together
- Vegetables 1 cup

NUTRITION FACTS

Calories: 380   Fat: 18.2 g   Carbs: 25 g   Protein: 28 g

The Total Protein intake is 74.3 grams of protein. I would have 1 scoop of protein after your workout making a grand total of 99.3.

9. Week 4 Yoga Workout

Yoga

Every day this week is a yoga day, and will be focused on comfortable stretches, releasing the tension and aches of the previous 3 weeks of exercise. Make sure these movements flow, and hold the positions for at least three breaths for each. Once you are done, switch back to the warm-up cross-leg position to rest. Also, be sure to get a Yoga mat, or at least do this on a comfortable floor.

I'll explain how to do the poses first time around. Breather is like a Rep but it lasts as long as you can hold an inhale and exhale. If you're still having trouble or are not sure if you're doing the stretches right, try a Google search.

Monday

Warm-up, or meditate, by sitting cross-legged on the floor. Make sure your back is straight and your hands are relaxed on your lap. Relax, close your eyes, and slowly breathe in and out as you bend your body left and right for 15 breaths. Do this after your wake-up water but before breakfast.

Cow and Cat pose – Stand on all fours. Cow pose arcs your back down, press shoulders away from head. Cat pose rounds your back, lowers your head, lifts belly and you try to see your thighs. Switch from Cow to Cat 5 times.

Downward Dog pose – Still on all fours, arc your back up to form a triangle or inverted V. Try to push your knees down and then back up. Hold, then rise and repeat 5 times.

Extended Side Angle – Lead with your right leg in a lunge, turn heel 45 degrees. With your right hand lose, reach and extend with your right over your head, making a straight line from heel to fingers. Hold for the usual 3 breaths, and then switch once to lean on your left leg.

Child's Pose – kneel down, lay back and face down as your hands stretch out. Keep your chest as close to your legs as possible. Simply relax and breathe.

Rest break of 1 minute

Downward Dog pose – repeat 5 times

Extended Side Angle – start left, then right. Hold for 3 breathers each.
Cow and Cat pose – switch 5 times

Child Pose – hold for 5 breathers.

Rest for 5 minutes, end session.

Walking

Walk 6000 steps today on top of your Yoga.

Nutrition

For the duration of this week, we'll be eating less protein. That means no meats unless it's a cheat meal, and that you'll have to eat a lot more fruits and veggies.

Upon Waking:

Have a long glass of warm water with lemon - either fresh lemon or pure lemon dripped in.

12 PM Breakfast – Meal One

- 1 x multivitamin
- An Orange
- Mixed with Green beans cut up

NUTRITION FACTS

Calories: 289   Fat: 4.4 g   Carbs: 34 g   Protein: 5.3 g

4 PM Lunch – Meal Two

- Fruit Salad Cup (Peach, Pear, Apricot, Pineapple, Cherry)
- Frozen Yogurt

NUTRITION FACTS
Calories: 275 Fat: 2.1g Carbs: 49.5g Protein: 21.3g

7 PM Dinner – Meal Three

- Smooth Peanut-Butter Sandwich (2 cups, 2 slices of bread)
- Apple

NUTRITION FACTS

Calories: 442 Fat: 18.3g Carbs: 60.3g Protein: 15.8

Total protein gain is 42.4 g. However, this week is about stretching muscles then building them. You need more protein when you work out because it converts to muscle. If you earn too much protein and don't work it off, you'll instead get fat, which is not what we want. That's why for your diet this week, abstain on eating meat and cups of protein.

Tuesday

Meditate cross-legged style for 15 breaths. Do this after the wake-up water but before breakfast.

<u>Yoga</u>

Mountain Pose – stand tall, feet together, shoulders relaxed. Each one of your 3 breathers, try to extend higher.

Tree Pose – arms raised then prayer, balance on one leg. Switch to next leg after 15 breathers.

Warrior Pose – stand 3-4 feet apart, bend forward leg 90 degrees, stay for 1 minute or 15 breathers before switching.

Pidgeon Pose – from a push-up position, kneel your left knee near shoulder. Lower down to forearms, allow right foot to be placed perfectly against the floor. Hold for 15 breathers and then switch legs.

Rest for 1 minute.

Pidgeon Pose – 15 breathers for each leg.

Tree Pose – 15 breathers for each leg.

Mountain Pose – 3 breathers, reach higher each time
Warrior Pose – 15 breathers for each leg.

Rest for 5 minutes, end session.

Walking

Walk 6000 steps today on top of your Yoga.

Nutrition

Upon Waking:

Have a long glass of warm water with lemon - either fresh lemon or pure lemon dripped in.

12 PM Breakfast – Meal One

- 1 x multivitamin
- An Orange
- Mixed with Green beans cut up

NUTRITION FACTS

Calories: 289   Fat: 4.4 g   Carbs: 34 g   Protein: 5.3 g

4 PM Lunch – Meal Two

- Fruit Salad Cup (Peach, Pear, Apricot, Pineapple, Cherry)
- Frozen Yogurt

NUTRITION FACTS
Calories: 275 Fat: 2.1g Carbs: 49.5g Protein: 21.3g

7 PM Dinner – Meal Three

- Smooth Peanut-Butter Sandwich (2 cups, 2 slices of bread)
- Apple

NUTRITION FACTS

Calories: 442 Fat: 18.3g Carbs: 60.3g Protein: 15.8

Total protein gain is 42.4 g.

Wednesday

Meditate cross-legged style for 15 breaths. Do this after wake-up water but before breakfast.

Yoga

Bridge Pose – lie on floor on your back with bent knees and arms flat on floor. Lift hips with feet in place as you exhale. Hold for 1 minute or 15 breathers.

Cobra Pose – lie face first on the floor, thumbs under shoulders and top of the feet on the floor slide. Push your body through thumb and index finger to rise upper body. Rinse and repeat 5 times.

Crow Pose – From Downward Dog position, move feet forward until the knees are touching the arms. Bend your elbows, stand on your toes, and rest knees against arms. Hold position for 10 breathers.

Seated Twist – Sit down with legs extended. Cross right foot over outside of left thigh and bend right knee with it pointed to ceiling. Place left elbow outside of right knee and right hand behind you on the floor. Twist your abdomen as far as you can, with your butt firm on the floor. Hold for a minute or 15 breathers before switching to the other side.

Rest for 1 minute.

Seated Twist – 15 breathers for each side.

Cobra Pose – Rise and fall 5 times.

Bridge Pose – Hold for 15 breathers.

Crow Pose – Hold for 10 breathers.

Walking

Walk 6000 steps today on top of your Yoga.

Nutrition

Upon Waking:

Have a long glass of warm water with lemon - either fresh lemon or pure lemon dripped in.

12 PM Breakfast – Meal One

- 1 x multivitamin
- An Orange
- Porridge Oats 30gram serving with 1 tbsp. honey

NUTRITION FACTS

Calories: 427 Fat: 8.2g   Carbs: 50.2 g Protein: 8.9 g

4 P.M - Lunch - Meal Two

- Full-Fat Cottage Cheese
- 1 cups Cashews
- 1 Apple

NUTRITION FACTS

Calories: 356   Fat: 17 g Carb: 9 g   Protein: 26 g

7 PM Dinner – Meal Three

- Canned Tomato Soup
- Full-Fat Cottage Cheese
- Saltine Crackers

NUTRITION FACTS

Calories: 292 Fat: 7.2g Carb: 41g Protein: 18.7g

Total protein gain is 53.6g. Remember not to eat any protein cups this week.

Thursday

Meditate cross-legged style for 15 breaths. Do this after wake-up water but before breakfast.

Yoga

Again, flow and hold the positions for three breaths for each. Once you are done, switch back to the warm-up cross-leg position to rest.

Cow and Cat pose – Switch from Cow to Cat 5 times.
Downward Dog pose – Hold and then switch 5 times
Extended Side Angle – switch legs after 3 breathers
Child's Pose – hold for 5 breaths

Rest break of 1 minute

Downward Dog pose – repeat 5 times

Extended Side Angle – switch legs after 3 breathers
Cow and Cat pose – switch 5 times

Child Pose – hold for 5 breathers.

Rest for 5 minutes, end session.

Walking

Walk 6000 steps today on top of your Yoga.

Nutrition

Upon Waking:

Have a long glass of warm water with lemon - either fresh lemon or pure lemon dripped in.

12 PM Breakfast – Meal One

- 1 x multivitamin
- An Orange
- Mixed with Green beans cut up

NUTRITION FACTS

Calories: 289   Fat: 4.4 g   Carbs: 34 g   Protein: 5.3 g

4 PM Lunch – Meal Two

- Fruit Salad Cup (Peach, Pear, Apricot, Pineapple, Cherry)
- Frozen Yogurt

NUTRITION FACTS
Calories: 275 Fat: 2.1 g Carbs: 49.5g Protein: 21.3g

7 PM Dinner – Meal Three

- Smooth Peanut-Butter Sandwich (2 cups, 2 slices of bread)
- Apple

NUTRITION FACTS

Calories: 442 Fat: 18.3g Carbs: 60.3g Protein: 15.8

Total protein gain is 42.4g.

Friday

Meditate cross-legged style for 15 breaths. Do this after wake-up water but before breakfast.

Seated Twist – 15 breathers for each side.
Pidgeon Pose – 15 breathers per leg.
Downward Dog – repeat 5 times.
Child Pose – hold for 5 breathers.

Rest for 1 minute.

Pidgeon Pose – 15 breathers per leg.
Downward Dog – repeat 5 times.
Seated Twist – 15 breathers for each side.

Child Pose – hold for 5 breathers.

Rest for 5 minutes. End session.

Walking

Walk 6000 steps today on top of your Yoga.

Nutrition

Upon Waking:

Have a long glass of warm water with lemon - either fresh lemon or pure lemon dripped in.

12 PM Breakfast – Meal One

- 1 x multivitamin
- An Orange
- Porridge Oats 30gram serving with 1 tbsp. honey

NUTRITION FACTS

Calories: 427 Fat: 8.2 g   Carbs: 50.2 g Protein: 8.9 g

4 PM Lunch – Meal Two

- Full-Fat Cottage Cheese
- 1 cups Cashews
- 1 Apple

NUTRITION FACTS

Calories: 356   Fat: 17 g Carb: 9 g   Protein: 26 g

7 PM Dinner – Meal Three

- Smooth Peanut-Butter Sandwich (2 cups, 2 slices of bread)
- Apple

NUTRITION FACTS

Calories: 442 Fat: 18.3g Carbs: 60.3g Protein: 15.8

Total protein gain is 50.7g

Saturday

Tree Pose – 15 breathers for each leg.

Extended Side Angle – switch legs between 3 breathers
Mountain Pose – 3 breathers, reach higher each time

Warrior Pose – 15 breathers for each leg.

Rest for 1 minute.

Mountain Pose – 3 breathers, reach higher each time.
Warrior Pose – 15 breathers for each leg.

Extended Side Angle – switch legs between 3 breathers.

Tree Pose – 15 breathers for each leg

Rest for 5 minutes. End session.

Walking

Walk 6000 steps today on top of your Yoga.

Nutrition

Upon Waking:

Have a long glass of warm water with lemon - either fresh lemon or pure lemon dripped in.

12 P.M - Breakfast - Meal One

- 1 x multivitamin
- An Orange
- Porridge Oats 30gram serving with 1 tbsp. honey

NUTRITION FACTS

Calories: 427 Fat: 8.2 g   Carbs: 50.2 g Protein: 8.9 g

4 P.M - Lunch - Meal Two

- Full-Fat Cottage Cheese
- 1 cups Cashews
- 1 Apple

NUTRITION FACTS

Calories: 356   Fat: 17 g Carb: 9 g   Protein: 26 g

7 PM Dinner

- Canned Tomato Soup
- Full-Fat Cottage Cheese
- Saltine Crackers

NUTRITION FACTS

Calories: 292 Fat: 7.2g Carb: 41g Protein: 18.7g

Total protein gain is 53.6g

Sunday - Rest and Nutrition

So we have reached the end of week 4. This was a lighter week, just to allow the body to regroup, to readjust your goals and to see and feel your progress. We are moving forward, even if you don't feel like it, or skipped a few days, reset your mind to do better this week.

For being so dedicated I've given you two cheat meals today, they can actually be wherever you want - Breakfast/Dinner, Breakfast/Lunch etc. It's important for us to kick back and enjoy our hard work and to indulge in the odd cake.

Today is all about chilling, eating well, having your cheat meal - which is anything of your choice. I've also added a sneaky scoop of ice cream with your protein shake for doing so well.

Of course, come tomorrow of this workout you'll need to step up and work just as hard as the first three weeks. But for now, you earned yourself a reward to relax. You don't have to stick to the regimented Intermittent Fasting rules, so today you can take a break.

Upon Waking:

Have a long glass of warm water with lemon - either fresh lemon or pure lemon dripped in.

Breakfast - Meal One

- 1 x multivitamin
- 1 x Whey Protein shake - with peanut butter, a banana and a scoop of ice cream
- 1 30gram x Bowl of Granola

NUTRITION FACTS

Calories: 561   Fat: 35.4 g   Carbs: 26.2 g   Protein: 30 g

Lunch - Meal Two

CHEAT MEAL - whatever you fancy!

Dinner - Meal

CHEAT MEAL - whatever you fancy!

10. Week 5 Weights Workout

It's back to weights again for your 5th week of intermittent fasting. This time we start with Back and Biceps for a change.

Monday - Back and Biceps

Once more with feeling – weights go!

Walk: 30 Minutes of cardio before breakfast. Burn the fat and get the body ready.

Weights: I would do this around 4-6 when you're strongest. Or straight after work before dinner.

Round 1

Increase the weight little by little with each set. 45 second between sets.

Exercise	Sets/Reps
CHIN-UP	1-2 sets of 20 reps (warm-up); 3 sets of 15, 12, 10 reps
Superset	
BARBELL CURL	3 sets of 15-20 reps

Round 2

Increase the weight little by little with each set.

Exercise	Sets/Reps
WIDE-GRIP REAR PULL-UP	3 sets of 20, 15, 10 reps
Superset	
DUMBBELL ALTERNATE BICEP CURL	3 sets of 15-20 reps

Round 3

Increase the weight little by little with each set.

Exercise	Sets/Reps
T-BAR ROW	3 sets of 20, 15, 10 reps
Superset	
INCLINE DUMBBELL CURL	3 sets of 15-20 rep

Nutrition

Upon Waking:

Have a long glass of warm water with lemon - either fresh lemon or pure lemon dripped in.

12 P.M - Breakfast - Meal One

- 1 x multivitamin
- 2 Whole Eggs Scrambled
- Mixed with Green beans cut up

NUTRITION FACTS

Calories: 409   Fat: 17.6 g   Carbs: 20.6 g   Protein: 16.3 g

4 P.M - Lunch - Meal Two

- Chicken Breast - With parsley, and bell peppers sliced up
- Vegetables - 1-2 cups

NUTRITION FACTS

Calories: 318   Fat: 15g   Carbs: 15g   Protein: 24g

7 PM - Dinner - Meal Three

- Tuna Steak
- Rocket and sliced Red Peppers
- Medium Sweet Potato

NUTRITION FACTS

Calories: 456   Fat: 17g Carbs: 29g   Protein: 28g

Tuesday - Abs/Cardio + Nutrition

Upon Waking:

Have a long glass of warm water with lemon - either fresh lemon or pure lemon dripped in.

Before Breakfast:

20 x Crunches x 3

25 twists x 3 each side

Run: 25-minute run (remember to warm up and down) Try to walk as much as possible, later on to from work or to a further station etc.

12 P.M - Breakfast - Meal One

- 1 x multivitamin
- 1 x Whey Protein shake - with peanut butter and a banana
- 1 30gram x Bowl of Granola

NUTRITION FACTS

Calories: 561   Fat: 30.4 g   Carbs: 26.2 g   Protein: 28 g

4 P.M - Lunch - Meal Two

- 1 x Medium sized Tuna Steak
- 1 x Cup Vegetables/salad

NUTRITION FACTS

Calories: 471   Fat: 33.2 g   Carbs: 17 g   Protein: 27 g

7 P.M - Dinner - Meal Three

- 2 Large Eggs Omelet with chopped green beans
- 2 Rice Cakes
- 1 x Peach

NUTRITION FACTS

Calories: 349   Fat: 14 g Carb: 25 g   Protein: 16 g

The Total Protein intake is 71 grams of protein. I would have 1 scoop of protein plus after your workout making a grand total of 96.

Wednesday - Chest and Triceps

Walk: 30 Minute brisk walk before breakfast - again breakfast is ideal.

Weights: As I said before breakfast or straight after work.

Round 1

Increase the weight little by little with each set. 45 second break between sets.

Exercise	Sets/Reps
BARBELL BENCH PRESS - MEDIUM GRIP	1-2 sets of 20 reps (warm-up); 3 sets of 15, 12, 10 reps
Superset	
LYING TRICEPS PRESS	3 sets of 15, 12, 10 reps

Round 2

Increase the weight little by little with each set.

Exercise	Sets/Reps
BARBELL INCLINE BENCH PRESS	3 sets of 15, 12, 10 reps
Superset	
TRICEPS PUSHDOWN	3 sets of 20, 15, 10 reps

Round 3

Increase the weight little by little with each set.

Exercise	Sets/Reps
DUMBBELL FLYES	3 sets of 15, 12, 10 reps
Superset	
CABLE ROPE OVERHEAD TRICEPS EXTENSION	3 sets of 20, 15, 10 reps

Nutrition

Upon Waking:

Have a long glass of warm water with lemon - either fresh lemon or pure lemon dripped in.

12 P.M - Breakfast - Meal One

- 1 x multivitamin
- 2 boiled eggs
- Porridge Oats 30gram serving with 1 tbsp. honey

NUTRITION FACTS

Calories: 409   Fat: 17.6 g   Carbs: 35.6 g   Protein: 20.3 g

4 P.M - Lunch - Meal Two

- Pork Chops 5 ounces- with cooked apple - cooked together
- Vegetables 1 cup

NUTRITION FACTS

Calories: 380   Fat: 18.2 g   Carbs: 25 g   Protein: 28 g

7 P.M - Dinner - Meal Three

- Full-Fat Cottage Cheese
- 1 cup Cashews
- 1 Apple
- 1 Banana

NUTRITION FACTS

Calories: 556   Fat: 17 g Carb: 59 g   Protein: 28 g

The Total Protein intake is 76.3 grams of protein. I would have 1 scoop of protein after your workout making a grand total of 101.3.

Thursday - Abs/Cardio + Nutrition

Upon Waking:

Have a long glass of warm water with lemon - either fresh lemon or pure lemon dripped in.

Run: 30-minute run before breakfast. I'd like you to get in a good 30-minute walk at the end of the day.

After work:

25 twists x 3 each side

Hold plank - 30 seconds x 3 (This helps strengthen your core body)

12 P.M - Breakfast - Meal One

- 1 x multivitamin
- 2 Whole Eggs Scrambled
- Mixed with Green beans cut up

NUTRITION FACTS

Calories: 409   Fat: 17.6 g   Carbs: 20.6 g   Protein: 16.3 g

4 P.M - Lunch - Meal Two

- Chicken Breast - With parsley, and bell peppers sliced up
- Steamed Broccoli

NUTRITION FACTS

Calories: 318   Fat: 15g   Carbs: 15g   Protein: 24g

7 PM - Dinner - Meal Three

- Tuna Steak
- Cucumber, tomatoes, Wild Rocket and Celery chunks

NUTRITION FACTS

Calories: 376   Fat: 17g Carbs: 9g   Protein: 27g

The Total Protein intake is 67.3 grams of protein. I would have 1 scoop of protein - 25grams - after your workout making a grand total of 92.3.

Notice how the carbs are minimal - except after your training. You can have carbs then, then stick with veg and fruit.

Friday - Legs and Calves

Walk: 25-minute walk early to work, or before work round the block - it's leg day and so need to do anything too hard.

<u>Round 1</u>

I would certainly do this work out after work, amongst your feeding time so you have energy to train and can replace energy. Warm up thoroughly. Increase the weight little by little with each set.

Exercise	Sets/Reps
BARBELL SQUAT	2 warm up light sets, 3 sets of 15, 12, 10 reps
STANDING LEG CURL	3 sets of 20, 15, 12 reps
SMITH MACHINE LEG PRESS	3 sets of 10 reps

Round 2

Increase the weight little by little with each set.

Exercise	Sets/Reps
DEADLIFT	3 sets of 15, 12, 10 reps
LEG EXTENSIONS	3 sets of 20, 15, 12 reps
LEG CURLS	3 sets of 10 reps

Round 3

Increase the weight little by little with each set.

Exercise	Sets/Reps
STANDING CALF RAISES	3 sets of 20, 15, 10 reps
SEATED CALF RAISE	3 sets of 15-20 reps

Nutrition

Upon Waking:

Have a long glass of warm water with lemon - either fresh lemon or pure lemon dripped in.

12 P.M - Breakfast - Meal One

- 1 x multivitamin
- 1 x Whey Protein shake - with peanut butter and a banana
- 1 30gram x Bowl of Granola

NUTRITION FACTS

Calories: 561   Fat: 30.4 g   Carbs: 26.2 g   Protein: 28 g

4 P.M - Lunch - Meal Two

- Greek Yogurt - High Protein
- 1 x Sliced Peach
- 2 cups Cashews

NUTRITION FACTS

Calories: 752   Fat: 34 g Carb: 18 g   Protein: 52 g

7 P.M - Dinner - Meal Three

- 1 x Medium sized Tuna Steak
- 1 x Cup Vegetables/salad
- 1 Medium sized Baked Potato

NUTRITION FACTS

Calories: 571   Fat: 33.2 g   Carbs: 80 g   Protein: 33 g

I've given you a huge carb dinner here after the leg workout and this will replenish your energy. Add a dab of butter too. The Total Protein intake is 113 grams of protein. I would have 1 scoop of protein plus after your workout making a grand total of 138.

Saturday - Abs/Cardio + Nutrition

Upon Waking:

Have a long glass of warm water with lemon - either fresh lemon or pure lemon dripped in.

Before Breakfast: - Ab Blast

20 x Crunches

25 x Twists

15 x sit-ups

20 x Crunches

25 x Twists

15 x sit-ups

20 x Crunches

25 x Twists

15 x sit-ups

Run: 30-minute run - during the morning.

12 P.M - Breakfast - Meal One

- 1 x multivitamin
- 1 Whole Egg
- 1 piece of salmon
- Oats 1/4 cup with 1 tbsp. honey

NUTRITION FACTS

Calories: 561   Fat: 30.4 g   Carbs: 20.2 g   Protein: 26.1 g

4 P.M - Lunch - Meal Two

- High Protein Frozen Yogurt
- Cashews 2 ounces
- 1 Apple

NUTRITION FACTS

Calories: 356   Fat: 17 g Carb: 9 g   Protein: 26 g

7 P.M - Dinner - Meal Four

- Pork Chops 5 ounces- with cooked apple - cooked together
- Vegetables 1 cup

NUTRITION FACTS

Calories: 380   Fat: 18.2 g   Carbs: 25 g   Protein: 28 g

The Total Protein intake is 80.1 grams of protein. I would have 1 scoop of protein after your workout making a grand total of 105.1.

Sunday - Rest

Another week, another well-earned rest. Feel free to have your cheat meal for lunch, again without worry about nutrition facts.

Upon Waking:

Have a long glass of warm water with lemon - either fresh lemon or pure lemon dripped in.

Breakfast - Meal One

- 1 x multivitamin
- 3 x scrambled eggs - with spinach
- 1 30gram x Bowl of Granola

NUTRITION FACTS

Calories: 561   Fat: 30.4 g   Carbs: 26.2 g   Protein: 26 g

Lunch - Meal Two

CHEAT MEAL - whatever you fancy!

7 P.M - Dinner - Meal Three

- 1 Cup x Full-Fat Cottage Cheese
- 1 x blob of peanut butter mixed in

NUTRITION FACTS

Calories: 371   Fat: 27 g Carb: 9 g   Protein: 24 g

11. Week 6 Cardio Workout

Monday - Cardio

Week 6 is all about cardio. So we allow the body time to recover from the weight training and now we focus on burning fat. We want to rev up your metabolism so we will be doing cardio in the morning before breakfast and we will making use of a pedometer that almost every smart phone has.

I want you to be doing 6000 steps a day this week on top of your cardio. That roughly equates to 1 hour of walking. Just work this into getting to and from work and a walk on your lunch break and it'll be done without even trying.

Here is a great routine for HIIT - High Intensity Interval Training. Let's ramp up the fat burning and get down to it!

Cardio

Do this 3 times. Go!

Three circuits: 10 reps per exercise. No rests.

Round One:

- **Burpees**
- **Press-ups**
- **Jumping Jacks**

- **Skipping rope: 3 minutes**

Rest 1 minute

Three circuits: 15 reps per exercise. No rest

Round Two:

- **Walking Lunges with kettlebell exchange underneath leg**
- **Star jumps**
- **High knees running on the spot**

- **Skipping rope: 3 minutes**

Rest 1 minute

Three circuits: 25 reps per exercise. No rest.

Round Three:

- **Pullups**
- **Box Jumps**
- **Star jumps**

- **Skipping rope: 3 minutes**

Rest 1 minute

Three circuits: 30 reps per move. No Rest

Round Four:

- **Alternate Side Lunges**
- **Dips**
- **Shadow boxing**

Nutrition

Upon Waking:

Have a long glass of warm water with lemon - either fresh lemon or pure lemon dripped in.

12 P.M - Breakfast - Meal One

- 1 x multivitamin
- 2 Whole Eggs Scrambled
- Mixed with Green beans cut up

NUTRITION FACTS

Calories: 409   Fat: 17.6 g   Carbs: 20.6 g   Protein: 16.3 g

4 P.M - Lunch - Meal Two

- 1 Can of Tuna Steak
- Red bell peppers, and low fat Coleslaw

NUTRITION FACTS

Calories: 386   Fat: 17g   Carbs: 17g   Protein: 27g

7 P.M - Dinner - Meal Three

- Chicken Breast - With parsley, and bell peppers sliced up
- Peas and Carrots

NUTRITION FACTS

Calories: 318   Fat: 15g   Carbs: 15g   Protein: 24g

The Total Protein intake is 67.3 grams of protein. I would have 1 scoop of protein - 25grams - after your workout making a grand total of 92.3.

Notice how the carbs are minimal - except after your training. You can have carbs then, then stick with veg and fruit.

Tuesday - Cardio

Before Breakfast:

Very simple, do about 5 minutes of stretches and then go for an early 30 minute run - outside or use the running machine in a gym.

Be sure to warm down.

Plus, remember your walking today - as much as you can.

Nutrition

Upon Waking:

Have a long glass of warm water with lemon - either fresh lemon or pure lemon dripped in.

12 P.M - Breakfast - Meal One

- 1 x multivitamin
- 1 x Whey Protein shake - with peanut butter and a banana
- 1 30gram x Bowl of Granola

NUTRITION FACTS

Calories: 561   Fat: 30.4 g   Carbs: 26.2 g   Protein: 28 g

4 P.M - Lunch - Meal Two

- 1 x Medium sized Tuna Steak
- 1 x Cup Vegetables/salad

NUTRITION FACTS

Calories: 471   Fat: 33.2 g   Carbs: 17 g   Protein: 27 g

7 PM - Dinner - Meal Three

- Tuna Steak
- Rocket and sliced Red Peppers

- Medium Sweet Potato

NUTRITION FACTS

Calories: 456   Fat: 17g Carbs: 29g   Protein: 28g

The Total Protein intake is 83 grams of protein. I would have 1 scoops of protein plus after your workout making a grand total of 108.

Wednesday - Cardio

Cardio

Do this 3 times. Go!

Three circuits: 10 reps per exercise. No rests.

Round One:

- **Burpees**
- **Press-ups**
- **Jumping Jacks**

- **Skipping rope: 3 minutes**

Rest 1 minute

Three circuits: 15 reps per exercise. No rest

Round Two:

- **Walking Lunges with kettlebell exchange underneath leg**
- **Star jumps**
- **High knees running on the spot**

- **Skipping rope: 3 minutes**

Rest 1 minute

Three circuits: 25 reps per exercise. No rest.

Round Three:

- **Pullups**
- **Box Jumps**
- **Star jumps**

- **Skipping rope: 3 minutes**

Rest 1 minute

Three circuits: 30 reps per move. No Rest

Round Four:

- **Alternate Side Lunges**
- **Dips**
- **Shadow boxing**

Nutrition

Upon Waking:

Have a long glass of warm water with lemon - either fresh lemon or pure lemon dripped in.

12 P.M - Breakfast - Meal One

- 1 x multivitamin
- 2 boiled eggs
- Porridge Oats 30gram serving with 1 tbsp. honey

NUTRITION FACTS

Calories: 409   Fat: 17.6 g   Carbs: 35.6 g   Protein: 20.3 g

4 P.M - Lunch - Meal Two

- Full-Fat Cottage Cheese
- 1 cup Cashews
- 1 Pear
- 1 Banana

NUTRITION FACTS

Calories: 566   Fat: 17 g Carb: 59 g   Protein: 28 g

7 P.M - Dinner - Meal Three

- Pork Chops 5 ounces- with cooked apple - cooked together
- Vegetables 1 cup

NUTRITION FACTS

Calories: 380   Fat: 18.2 g   Carbs: 25 g   Protein: 28 g

The Total Protein intake is 76.3 grams of protein. I would have 1 scoop of protein after your workout making a grand total of 101.3.

Thursday - Cardio

Before Breakfast:

Very simple, do about 5 minutes of stretches and then go for an early 25 minutes of spinning or a bike ride - outside or use the running machine in a gym.

Or just stick to the pavement and do a 30 minute run.

Be sure to warm down.

Nutrition

Upon Waking:

Have a long glass of warm water with lemon - either fresh lemon or pure lemon dripped in.

12 P.M - Breakfast - Meal One

- 1 x multivitamin
- 1 x Whey Protein shake - with peanut butter and a banana
- 1 30gram x Bowl of Granola

NUTRITION FACTS

Calories: 561   Fat: 30.4 g   Carbs: 26.2 g   Protein: 28 g

4 P.M Lunch - Meal Two

- 1 x can of Tuna Steak
- Rocket and Beetroot

NUTRITION FACTS

Calories: 471   Fat: 33.2 g   Carbs: 17 g   Protein: 27 g

7 P.M Dinner - Meal Three

- Chicken Breast - With parsley, and bell peppers sliced up
- Steamed Broccoli

NUTRITION FACTS

Calories: 318   Fat: 15g   Carbs: 15g   Protein: 24g

The Total Protein intake is 79 grams of protein. I would have 1 scoops of protein plus after your workout making a grand total of 104.

Friday - Cardio

Cardio

Do this 3 times. Go!

Three circuits: 10 reps per exercise. No rests.

Round One:

- **Burpees**
- **Press-ups**
- **Jumping Jacks**

- **Skipping rope: 3 minutes**

Rest 1 minute

Three circuits: 15 reps per exercise. No rest

Round Two:

- **Walking Lunges with kettlebell exchange underneath leg**
- **Star jumps**
- **High knees running on the spot**

- **Skipping rope: 3 minutes**

Rest 1 minute

Three circuits: 25 reps per exercise. No rest.

Round Three:

- **Pullups**
- **Box Jumps**
- **Star jumps**

- **Skipping rope: 3 minutes**

Rest 1 minute

Three circuits: 30 reps per move. No Rest

Round Four:

- **Alternate Side Lunges**
- **Dips**
- **Shadow boxing**

Nutrition

Upon Waking:

Have a long glass of warm water with lemon - either fresh lemon or pure lemon dripped in.

12 P.M - Breakfast - Meal One

- 1 x multivitamin
- 2 Whole Eggs Scrambled
- Mixed with Green beans cut up

NUTRITION FACTS

Calories: 409   Fat: 17.6 g   Carbs: 20.6 g   Protein: 16.3 g

4 P.M Lunch - Meal Two

- 1 x Medium sized Tuna Steak
- 1 x Cup Vegetables/salad
- 1 Medium sized Baked Potato

NUTRITION FACTS

Calories: 571   Fat: 33.2 g   Carbs: 80 g   Protein: 33 g

7 P.M - Dinner - Meal Three

- Chicken Breast - With parsley, and bell peppers sliced up
- Sprouts - cooked and mashed - add pepper and soft cheese - mash up

NUTRITION FACTS

Calories: 418   Fat: 15g   Carbs: 28g   Protein: 29g

The Total Protein intake is 78.3 grams of protein. I would have 1 scoop of protein - 25grams - after your workout making a grand total of 103.3.

Saturday - Cardio

<u>Before Breakfast</u>

1 hour of swimming - or 1 x 45 minute insanity workout.

In terms of swimming I want to mix it up, this is also very low impact, your muscles could probably do with something relaxing. Try to put in lengths and keep moving.

Again warming up and cooling down is very important.

Nutrition

Upon Waking:

Have a long glass of warm water with lemon - either fresh lemon or pure lemon dripped in.

12 P.M - Breakfast - Meal One

- 1 x multivitamin
- 2 boiled eggs
- Porridge Oats 30gram serving with 1 tbsp. honey

NUTRITION FACTS

Calories: 409   Fat: 17.6 g   Carbs: 35.6 g   Protein: 20.3 g

4 P.M - Lunch - Meal Two

- Full-Fat Cottage Cheese
- 1 cups Cashews
- 1 Apple

NUTRITION FACTS

Calories: 356   Fat: 17 g   Carb: 9 g   Protein: 26 g

7 P.M - Dinner - Meal Three

- Pork Chops 5 ounces- with cooked apple - cooked together
- Vegetables 1 cup

NUTRITION FACTS

Calories: 380   Fat: 18.2 g   Carbs: 25 g   Protein: 28 g

The Total Protein intake is 74.3 grams of protein. I would have 1 scoop of protein after your workout making a grand total of 99.3.

Sunday - Rest and Nutrition

We've reached Week 2 of the workout! You're probably starting to notice the changes on your stomach becoming a set of abs, and the muscles on your arms and legs stating to form. But for now, let's give them a much needed breather, for today is your break day. After all those cardio workouts, your heart certainly needs it.

Like last week, you're free to have your cheat meal and lax eating times.

Upon Waking:

Have a long glass of warm water with lemon - either fresh lemon or pure lemon dripped in.

Breakfast - Meal One

- 1 x multivitamin
- 3 x scrambled eggs - with spinach
- 1 30gram x Bowl of Granola

NUTRITION FACTS

Calories: 561   Fat: 30.4 g   Carbs: 26.2 g   Protein: 26 g

Lunch - Meal Two

CHEAT MEAL - whatever you fancy!

7 P.M - Dinner - Meal Three

- 1 Cup x Full-Fat Cottage Cheese
- 1 x blob of peanut butter mixed in

NUTRITION FACTS

Calories: 371   Fat: 27 g Carb: 9 g   Protein: 24 g

12. Week 7 Yoga Workout

Monday

We are back to Yoga for week 7. Warm-up, or meditate, by sitting cross-legged on the floor. Make sure your back is straight and your hands are relaxed on your lap. Relax, close your eyes, and slowly breathe in and out as you bend your body left and right for 15 breaths. Do this after your wake-up water but before breakfast.

Yoga

Make sure these movements flow, and hold the positions for at least three breaths for each. Once you are done, switch back to the warm-up cross-leg position to rest. Also, be sure to get a Yoga mat, or at least do this on a comfortable floor.

I'll explain how to do the poses first time around. Breather is like a Rep but it lasts as long as you can hold an inhale and exhale. If you're still having trouble or are not sure if you're doing the stretches right, try a Google search.

Cow and Cat pose – Stand on all fours. Cow pose arcs your back down, press shoulders away from head. Cat pose rounds your back, lowers your head, lifts belly and you try to see your thighs. Switch from Cow to Cat 5 times.

Downward Dog pose – Still on all fours, arc your back up to form a triangle or inverted V. Try to push your knees down and then back up. Hold, then rise and repeat 5 times.

Extended Side Angle – Lead with your right leg in a lunge, turn heel 45 degrees. With your right hand lose, reach and extend with your right over your head, making a straight line from heel to fingers. Hold for the usual 3 breaths, and then switch once to lean on your left leg.

Child's Pose – kneel down, lay back and face down as your hands stretch out. Keep your chest as close to your legs as possible. Simply relax and breathe.

Rest break of 1 minute

Downward Dog pose – repeat 5 times

Extended Side Angle – start left, then right. Hold for 3 breathers each.
Cow and Cat pose – switch 5 times

Child Pose – hold for 5 breathers.

Rest for 5 minutes, end session.

Nutrition

For the duration of this week, we'll be eating less protein. That means no meats unless it's a cheat meal, and that you'll have to eat a lot more fruits and veggies.

Upon Waking:

Have a long glass of warm water with lemon - either fresh lemon or pure lemon dripped in.

12 PM Breakfast – Meal One

- 1 x multivitamin
- An Orange
- Mixed with Green beans cut up

NUTRITION FACTS

Calories: 289   Fat: 4.4 g   Carbs: 34 g   Protein: 5.3 g

4 PM Lunch – Meal Two

- Fruit Salad Cup (Peach, Pear, Apricot, Pineapple, Cherry)
- Frozen Yogurt

NUTRITION FACTS
Calories: 275 Fat: 2.1g Carbs: 49.5g Protein: 21.3g

7 PM Dinner – Meal Three

- Smooth Peanut-Butter Sandwich (2 cups, 2 slices of bread)
- Apple

NUTRITION FACTS

Calories: 442 Fat: 18.3g Carbs: 60.3g Protein: 15.8

Total protein gain is 42.4 g. However, this week is about stretching muscles then building them. You need more protein when you work out because it converts to muscle. If you earn too much protein and don't work it off, you'll instead get fat, which is not what we want. That's why for your diet this week, abstain on eating meat and cups of protein.

Tuesday

Meditate cross-legged style for 15 breaths. Do this after the wake-up water but before breakfast.

Yoga

Mountain Pose – stand tall, feet together, shoulders relaxed. Each one of your 3 breathers, try to extend higher.

Tree Pose – arms raised then prayer, balance on one leg. Switch to next leg after 15 breathers.

Warrior Pose – stand 3-4 feet apart, bend forward leg 90 degrees, stay for 1 minute or 15 breathers before switching.

Pidgeon Pose – from a push-up position, kneel your left knee near shoulder. Lower down to forearms, allow right foot to be placed perfectly against the floor. Hold for 15 breathers and then switch legs.

Rest for 1 minute.

Pidgeon Pose – 15 breathers for each leg.

Tree Pose – 15 breathers for each leg.

Mountain Pose – 3 breathers, reach higher each time
Warrior Pose – 15 breathers for each leg.

Rest for 5 minutes, end session.

Nutrition

Upon Waking:

Have a long glass of warm water with lemon - either fresh lemon or pure lemon dripped in.

12 PM Breakfast – Meal One

- 1 x multivitamin
- An Orange
- Mixed with Green beans cut up

NUTRITION FACTS

Calories: 289   Fat: 4.4 g   Carbs: 34 g   Protein: 5.3 g

4 PM Lunch – Meal Two

- Fruit Salad Cup (Peach, Pear, Apricot, Pineapple, Cherry)
- Frozen Yogurt

NUTRITION FACTS
Calories: 275 Fat: 2.1g Carbs: 49.5g Protein: 21.3g

7 PM Dinner – Meal Three

- Smooth Peanut-Butter Sandwich (2 cups, 2 slices of bread)
- Apple

NUTRITION FACTS

Calories: 442 Fat: 18.3g Carbs: 60.3g Protein: 15.8

Total protein gain is 42.4 g.

Wednesday

Meditate cross-legged style for 15 breaths. Do this after wake-up water but before breakfast.

<u>Yoga</u>

Bridge Pose – lie on floor on your back with bent knees and arms flat on floor. Lift hips with feet in place as you exhale. Hold for 1 minute or 15 breathers.

Cobra Pose – lie face first on the floor, thumbs under shoulders and top of the feet on the floor slide. Push your body through thumb and index finger to rise upper body. Rinse and repeat 5 times.

Crow Pose – From Downward Dog position, move feet forward until the knees are touching the arms. Bend your elbows, stand on your toes, and rest knees against arms. Hold position for 10 breathers.

Seated Twist – Sit down with legs extended. Cross right foot over outside of left thigh and bend right knee with it pointed to ceiling. Place left elbow outside of right knee and right hand behind you on the floor. Twist your abdomen as far as you can, with your butt firm on the floor. Hold for a minute or 15 breathers before switching to the other side.

Rest for 1 minute.

Seated Twist – 15 breathers for each side.

Cobra Pose – Rise and fall 5 times.

Bridge Pose – Hold for 15 breathers.

Crow Pose – Hold for 10 breathers.

Nutrition

Upon Waking:

Have a long glass of warm water with lemon - either fresh lemon or pure lemon dripped in.

12 PM Breakfast – Meal One

- 1 x multivitamin
- An Orange
- Porridge Oats 30gram serving with 1 tbsp. honey

NUTRITION FACTS

Calories: 427 Fat: 8.2g   Carbs: 50.2 g Protein: 8.9 g

4 P.M - Lunch - Meal Two

- Full-Fat Cottage Cheese
- 1 cups Cashews
- 1 Apple

NUTRITION FACTS

Calories: 356   Fat: 17 g Carb: 9 g   Protein: 26 g

7 PM Dinner – Meal Three

- Canned Tomato Soup
- Full-Fat Cottage Cheese
- Saltine Crackers

NUTRITION FACTS

Calories: 292 Fat: 7.2g Carb: 41g Protein: 18.7g

Total protein gain is 53.6g. Remember not to eat any protein cups this week.

Thursday

Meditate cross-legged style for 15 breaths. Do this after wake-up water but before breakfast.

<u>Yoga</u>

Again, flow and hold the positions for three breaths for each. Once you are done, switch back to the warm-up cross-leg position to rest.

Cow and Cat pose – Switch from Cow to Cat 5 times.
Downward Dog pose – Hold and then switch 5 times
Extended Side Angle – switch legs after 3 breathers
Child's Pose – hold for 5 breaths

Rest break of 1 minute

Downward Dog pose – repeat 5 times

Extended Side Angle – switch legs after 3 breathers
Cow and Cat pose – switch 5 times

Child Pose – hold for 5 breathers.

Rest for 5 minutes, end session.

Nutrition

Upon Waking:

Have a long glass of warm water with lemon - either fresh lemon or pure lemon dripped in.

12 PM Breakfast – Meal One

- 1 x multivitamin
- An Orange
- Mixed with Green beans cut up

NUTRITION FACTS

Calories: 289   Fat: 4.4 g   Carbs: 34 g   Protein: 5.3 g

4 PM Lunch – Meal Two

- Fruit Salad Cup (Peach, Pear, Apricot, Pineapple, Cherry)
- Frozen Yogurt

NUTRITION FACTS
Calories: 275 Fat: 2.1 g Carbs: 49.5g Protein: 21.3g

7 PM Dinner – Meal Three

- Smooth Peanut-Butter Sandwich (2 cups, 2 slices of bread)
- Apple

NUTRITION FACTS

Calories: 442 Fat: 18.3g Carbs: 60.3g Protein: 15.8

Total protein gain is 42.4g.

Friday

Meditate cross-legged style for 15 breaths. Do this after wake-up water but before breakfast.

Seated Twist – 15 breathers for each side.
Pidgeon Pose – 15 breathers per leg.
Downward Dog – repeat 5 times.
Child Pose – hold for 5 breathers.

Rest for 1 minute.

Pidgeon Pose – 15 breathers per leg.
Downward Dog – repeat 5 times.
Seated Twist – 15 breathers for each side.

Child Pose – hold for 5 breathers.

Rest for 5 minutes. End session.

Nutrition

Upon Waking:

Have a long glass of warm water with lemon - either fresh lemon or pure lemon dripped in.

12 PM Breakfast – Meal One

- 1 x multivitamin
- An Orange
- Porridge Oats 30gram serving with 1 tbsp. honey

NUTRITION FACTS

Calories: 427 Fat: 8.2 g   Carbs: 50.2 g Protein: 8.9 g

4 PM Lunch – Meal Two

- Full-Fat Cottage Cheese
- 1 cups Cashews
- 1 Apple

NUTRITION FACTS

Calories: 356   Fat: 17 g Carb: 9 g   Protein: 26 g

7 PM Dinner – Meal Three

- Smooth Peanut-Butter Sandwich (2 cups, 2 slices of bread)

- Apple

NUTRITION FACTS

Calories: 442 Fat: 18.3g Carbs: 60.3g Protein: 15.8

Total protein gain is 50.7g

Saturday

Tree Pose – 15 breathers for each leg.

Extended Side Angle – switch legs between 3 breathers
Mountain Pose – 3 breathers, reach higher each time

Warrior Pose – 15 breathers for each leg.

Rest for 1 minute.

Mountain Pose – 3 breathers, reach higher each time.
Warrior Pose – 15 breathers for each leg.

Extended Side Angle – switch legs between 3 breathers.

Tree Pose – 15 breathers for each leg

Rest for 5 minutes. End session.

Nutrition

Upon Waking:

Have a long glass of warm water with lemon - either fresh lemon or pure lemon dripped in.

12 P.M - Breakfast - Meal One

- 1 x multivitamin
- An Orange
- Porridge Oats 30gram serving with 1 tbsp. honey

NUTRITION FACTS

Calories: 427 Fat: 8.2 g   Carbs: 50.2 g Protein: 8.9 g

4 P.M - Lunch - Meal Two

- Full-Fat Cottage Cheese
- 1 cups Cashews
- 1 Apple

NUTRITION FACTS

Calories: 356   Fat: 17 g Carb: 9 g   Protein: 26 g

7 PM Dinner

- Canned Tomato Soup
- Full-Fat Cottage Cheese
- Saltine Crackers

NUTRITION FACTS

Calories: 292 Fat: 7.2g Carb: 41g Protein: 18.7g

Total protein gain is 53.6g

Sunday - Rest and Nutrition

So we have reached the end of week 3. I hope you feel tired, and achy but more importantly feel like you're making progress, slimming down, looking great and feeling great. You are now half-way there, now!

For being so dedicated I've given you two cheat meals today, they can actually be wherever you want - Breakfast/Dinner, Breakfast/Lunch etc. It's important for us to kick back and enjoy our hard work and to indulge in the odd cake.

Today is all about chilling, eating well, having your cheat meal - which is anything of your choice. I've also added a sneaky scoop of ice cream with your protein shake for doing so well.

Of course, come tomorrow of this workout you'll need to step up and work just as hard as the first three weeks. But for now, you earned yourself a reward to relax. You don't have to stick to the regimented Intermittent Fasting rules, so today you can take a break.

Upon Waking:

Have a long glass of warm water with lemon - either fresh lemon or pure lemon dripped in.

Breakfast - Meal One

- 1 x multivitamin
- 1 x Whey Protein shake - with peanut butter, a banana and a scoop of ice cream
- 1 30gram x Bowl of Granola

NUTRITION FACTS

Calories: 561   Fat: 35.4 g   Carbs: 26.2 g   Protein: 30 g

Lunch - Meal Two

CHEAT MEAL - whatever you fancy!

Dinner - Meal

CHEAT MEAL - whatever you fancy!

13. Week 8 Weights Workout

Week eight begins and it's back to weights. We will train one day on weights and the next day off.

So let's go back to legs. Fantastic for building overall strength and conditioning - let's go.

Monday - Legs and Calves

Walk: 25-minute walk early to work, or before work round the block - it's leg day and so don't need to do anything too hard.

Round 1

I would certainly do this work out after work, amongst your feeding time so you have energy to train and can replace energy. Warm up thoroughly. Increase the weight little by little with each set.

Exercise	Sets/Reps
BARBELL SQUAT	2 warm up light sets, 3 sets of 12, 10, 8 reps
STANDING LEG CURL	3 sets of 15, 12, 10 reps
SMITH MACHINE LEG PRESS	3 sets of 8 reps

Do the Barbell Squat separately, and Superset the Standing Leg Curl and Leg Press

Round 2

Increase the weight little by little with each set.

Exercise	Sets/Reps
DEADLIFT	3 sets of 12, 10, 8 reps
LEG EXTENSIONS	3 sets of 15, 12, 10 reps
LEG CURLS	3 sets of 10 reps

Do the Deadlift separately, and Superset the Leg Extensions and Leg Curls

Round 3

Increase the weight little by little with each set.

Exercise	Sets/Reps
STANDING CALF RAISES	3 sets of 12, 10, 8 reps
Superset	
SEATED CALF RAISE	3 sets of 12-15 reps

Nutrition

Upon Waking:

Have a long glass of warm water with lemon - either fresh lemon or pure lemon dripped in.

12 P.M - Breakfast - Meal One

- 1 x multivitamin
- 2 Whole Eggs Scrambled
- Mixed with Green beans cut up

NUTRITION FACTS

Calories: 409   Fat: 17.6 g   Carbs: 20.6 g   Protein: 16.3 g

4 P.M - Lunch - Meal Two

- Chicken Breast - With parsley, and bell peppers sliced up
- Vegetables - 1-2 cups

NUTRITION FACTS

Calories: 318   Fat: 15g   Carbs: 15g   Protein: 24g

7 PM - Dinner - Meal Three

- Tuna Steak
- Rocket and sliced Red Peppers
- Medium Sweet Potato

NUTRITION FACTS

Calories: 456   Fat: 17g Carbs: 29g   Protein: 28g

The Total Protein intake is 68.3 grams of protein. I would have 1 scoop of protein - 25grams - after your workout making a grand total of 93.3.

Notice how the carbs are minimal - except after your training. You can have carbs then, then stick with veg and fruit.

Tuesday - Abs/Cardio + Nutrition

Upon Waking:

Have a long glass of warm water with lemon - either fresh lemon or pure lemon dripped in.

Before Breakfast: These can be done later in the day

3 sets- 20 Crunches each set

3 sets- 25 Standing Twists each direction

3 sets- 20 Side-Lying Leg Lifts each direction

Run: Again, do this later in the day, at least after the first meal.

25-minute run (remember to warm up and down)
Try to walk as much as possible, later on to from work or to a further station etc.

12 P.M - Breakfast - Meal One

- 1 x multivitamin
- 1 x Whey Protein shake - with peanut butter and a banana
- 1 30gram x Bowl of Granola

NUTRITION FACTS

Calories: 561   Fat: 30.4 g   Carbs: 26.2 g   Protein: 28 g

4 P.M - Lunch - Meal Two

- 1 x Medium sized Tuna Steak
- 1 x Cup Vegetables/salad

NUTRITION FACTS

Calories: 471   Fat: 33.2 g   Carbs: 17 g   Protein: 27

7 P.M - Dinner - Meal Three

- 2 Large Eggs Omelette with chopped green beans
- 2 Rice Cakes
- 1 x Peach

NUTRITION FACTS

Calories: 349   Fat: 14 g Carb: 25 g   Protein: 16 g

The Total Protein intake is 71 grams of protein. I would have 1 scoops of protein plus after your workout making a grand total of 96.

Wednesday - Chest and Triceps

Walk: 30 Minute brisk walk before breakfast - again breakfast is ideal.

Weights- Mid-afternoon is best.

Round 1

Increase the weight little by little with each set. 45 second break between sets.

Exercise	Sets/Reps
BARBELL BENCH PRESS - MEDIUM GRIP	1-2 sets of 15 reps (warm-up); 3 sets of 12, 10, 8 reps
Superset	
LYING TRICEPS PRESS	3 sets of 15, 12, 10 reps

Superset the Bench Press and Triceps Press

Round 2

Increase the weight little by little with each set.

Exercise	Sets/Reps
BARBELL INCLINE BENCH PRESS	3 sets of 12, 10, 8 reps
Superset	
TRICEPS PUSHDOWN	3 sets of 15, 12, 10 reps

Superset the Incline Bench Press and Triceps Pushdown

Round 3

Increase the weight little by little with each set.

Exercise	Sets/Reps
DUMBBELL FLYS	3 sets of 12, 10, 8 reps
Superset	
CABLE ROPE OVERHEAD TRICEPS EXTENSION	3 sets of 15, 12, 8 reps

Superset the Flies and Triceps Overhead Pulls

You can add a set of Push Ups at the end

Nutrition

Upon Waking:

Have a long glass of warm water with lemon - either fresh lemon or pure lemon dripped in.

12 P.M - Breakfast - Meal One

- 1 x multivitamin
- 2 boiled eggs
- Porridge Oats 30gram serving with 1 tbsp. honey

NUTRITION FACTS

Calories: 409   Fat: 17.6 g   Carbs: 35.6 g   Protein: 20.3 g

4 P.M - Lunch - Meal Two

- Pork Chops 5 ounces- with cooked apple - cooked together
- Vegetables 1 cup

NUTRITION FACTS

Calories: 380   Fat: 18.2 g   Carbs: 25 g   Protein: 28 g

7 P.M - Dinner - Meal Three

- Full-Fat Cottage Cheese
- 1 cup Cashews
- 1 Apple
- 1 Banana

NUTRITION FACTS

Calories: 556   Fat: 17 g Carb: 59 g   Protein: 28 g

The Total Protein intake is 76.3 grams of protein. I would have 1 scoop of protein after your workout making a grand total of 101.3.

Thursday - Abs/Cardio + Nutrition

Upon Waking:

Have a long glass of warm water with lemon - either fresh lemon or pure lemon dripped in.

Run: 30-minute run. I'd like you to get in a good 30-minute walk at the end of the day.

After work:

3 sets of 30 Twists each side

3 set of Side Bends each side- if too easy, add a 5-10 pound dumbbell

4 sets of Hold plank – 30 seconds each

12 P.M - Breakfast - Meal One

- 1 x multivitamin
- 2 Whole Eggs Scrambled
- Mixed with Green beans cut up

NUTRITION FACTS

Calories: 409   Fat: 17.6 g   Carbs: 20.6 g   Protein: 16.3 g

4 P.M - Lunch - Meal Two

- Chicken Breast - With parsley, and bell peppers sliced up
- Steamed Broccoli

NUTRITION FACTS

Calories: 318   Fat: 15g   Carbs: 15g   Protein: 24g

7 PM - Dinner - Meal Three

- Tuna Steak
- Cucumber, tomatoes, Wild Rocket and Celery chunks

NUTRITION FACTS

Calories: 376   Fat: 17g   Carbs: 9g   Protein: 27g

The Total Protein intake is 67.3 grams of protein. I would have 1 scoop of protein - 25grams - after your workout making a grand total of 92.3.

Notice how the carbs are minimal - except after your training. You can have carbs then, then stick with veg and fruit.

Friday - Back and Biceps

Walk: 30 Minutes of cardio before breakfast. We want to burn fat before anything else and get the body prepared for the day.

Round 1

Increase the weight little by little with each set. 45 second between sets.

Exercise	Sets/Reps
CHIN-UP	1-2 sets of 15 reps (warm-up); 3 sets of 12, 10, 8 reps
Superset	
BARBELL CURL	3 sets of 10-12 reps

If you cannot do many (or any) Chin-Ups, then stand on a stool to support some of your body weight. Hang down, and do the Chin-Up, pulling as hard as you can to pull up to the bar, and supporting as little of your weight on one foot.

Superset the Chin-Ups with the Barbell Curls- do one Chin-Up set, then a Barbell set, then repeat until finished.

Round 2

Increase the weight little by little with each set.

Exercise	Sets/Reps
WIDE-GRIP REAR PULL-UP	3 sets of 15, 12, 10 reps
Superset	
DUMBBELL ALTERNATE BICEP CURL	3 sets of 10-12 reps

Same as above if you cannot do many (or any) Pull-Ups.

Superset the Pull-Up sets with the Dumbbell Biceps Curls.

Round 3

Increase the weight little by little with each set.

Exercise	Sets/Reps
T-BAR ROW	3 sets of 15, 12, 8 reps
Superset	
INCLINE DUMBBELL REVERSE CURL	3 sets of 10-12 rep

Superset the Rows with the Dumbbell Reverse Curls. Reverse Curl means that your hands are facing away as you flex your elbow.

Nutrition

Upon Waking:

Have a long glass of warm water with lemon - either fresh lemon or pure lemon dripped in.

12 P.M - Breakfast - Meal One

- 1 x multivitamin
- 1 x Whey Protein shake - with peanut butter and a banana
- 1 30gram x Bowl of Granola

NUTRITION FACTS

Calories: 561   Fat: 30.4 g   Carbs: 26.2 g   Protein: 28 g

4 P.M - Lunch - Meal Two

- Greek Yogurt - High Protein
- 1 x Sliced Peach
- 2 cups Cashews

NUTRITION FACTS

Calories: 752   Fat: 34 g Carb: 18 g   Protein: 52 g

7 P.M - Dinner - Meal Three

- 1 x Medium sized Tuna Steak
- 1 x Cup Vegetables/salad
- 1 Medium sized Baked Potato

NUTRITION FACTS

Calories: 571   Fat: 33.2 g   Carbs: 80 g   Protein: 33 g

I've given you a huge carb dinner here after the leg workout and this will replenish your energy. Add a dab of butter too. The Total Protein intake is 113 grams of protein. I would have 1 scoops of protein plus after your workout making a grand total of 138.

Saturday - Abs/Cardio + Nutrition

Upon Waking:

Have a long glass of warm water with lemon - either fresh lemon or pure lemon dripped in.

Before Breakfast: - Ab Blast

20 x Crunches

25 x Twists

15 x sit-ups

20 x Crunches

25 x Twists

15 x sit-ups

20 x Crunches

25 x Twists

15 x sit-ups

Run: 30 minute run - during the morning.

12 P.M - Breakfast - Meal One

- 1 x multivitamin
- 1 Whole Egg
- 1 piece of salmon
- Oats 1/4 cup with 1 tbsp. honey

NUTRITION FACTS

Calories: 561   Fat: 30.4 g   Carbs: 20.2 g   Protein: 26.1 g

4 P.M - Lunch - Meal Two

- High Protein Frozen Yogurt
- Cashews 2 ounces
- 1 Apple

NUTRITION FACTS

Calories: 356   Fat: 17 g   Carb: 9 g   Protein: 26 g

7 P.M - Dinner - Meal Four

- Pork Chops 5 ounces- with cooked apple - cooked together
- Vegetables 1 cup

NUTRITION FACTS

Calories: 380   Fat: 18.2 g   Carbs: 25 g   Protein: 28 g

The Total Protein intake is 80.1 grams of protein. I would have 1 scoop of protein after your workout making a grand total of 105.1.

Sunday - Rest

So we've made it to our rest day - well done for an epic week 1 of workouts! You should be feeling good, a little achy maybe, but you got through it. Did you miss any workouts? If so, it doesn't matter, let's go one better this coming week. It's about progression.

So today is all about chilling, eating well, having your cheat meal - which is anything of your choice. Also it's Sunday so you don't need to follow the strict eating times if you want a break. Not that it should ever feel a chore, but having breakfast at the old breakfast time never hurt anyone on a Sunday.

Upon Waking:

Have a long glass of warm water with lemon - either fresh lemon or pure lemon dripped in.

Breakfast - Meal One

- 1 x multivitamin
- 3 x scrambled eggs - with spinach
- 1 30gram x Bowl of Granola

NUTRITION FACTS

Calories: 561   Fat: 30.4 g   Carbs: 26.2 g   Protein: 26 g

Lunch - Meal Two

CHEAT MEAL - whatever you fancy!

7 P.M - Dinner - Meal Three

- 1 Cup x Full-Fat Cottage Cheese
- 1 x blob of peanut butter mixed in

NUTRITION FACTS

Calories: 371   Fat: 27 g Carb: 9 g   Protein: 24 g

For future cheat meals, I'm not going into your exact macros here. Eat well and enjoy yourself until tomorrow.

14. Week 9 Workout Cardio

Monday - Cardio

Week 9 is all about intense cardio. Since we worked hard on weights, we're going to work harder on burning fat. On top of longer sets, this time you'll have to make 10000 steps a day. That's an extra 30mins to 1 hour of walking.

Cardio

Do this 3 times. Go!

Three circuits: 10 reps per exercise. No rests.

Round One:

- **Burpees**
- **Press-ups**
- **Jumping Jacks**

- **Skipping rope: 5 minutes**

Rest 1 minute

Three circuits: 20 reps per exercise. No rest

Round Two:

- **Walking Lunges with kettlebell exchange underneath leg**
- **Star jumps**
- **High knees running on the spot**

- **Skipping rope: 5 minutes**

Rest 1 minute

Three circuits: 30 reps per exercise. No rest.

Round Three:

- **Pullups**
- **Box Jumps**
- **Star jumps**
- **Skipping rope: 5 minutes**

Rest 1 minute

Three circuits: 40 reps per move. No Rest

Round Four:

- **Alternate Side Lunges**
- **Dips**
- **Shadow boxing**

Nutrition

Upon Waking:

Have a long glass of warm water with lemon - either fresh lemon or pure lemon dripped in.

12 P.M - Breakfast - Meal One

- 1 x multivitamin
- 2 Whole Eggs Scrambled
- Mixed with Green beans cut up

NUTRITION FACTS

Calories: 409   Fat: 17.6 g   Carbs: 20.6 g   Protein: 16.3 g

4 P.M - Lunch - Meal Two

- 1 Can of Tuna Steak
- Red bell peppers, and low fat Coleslaw

NUTRITION FACTS

Calories: 386   Fat: 17g   Carbs: 17g   Protein: 27g

7 P.M - Dinner - Meal Three

- Chicken Breast - With parsley, and bell peppers sliced up
- Peas and Carrots

NUTRITION FACTS

Calories: 318   Fat: 15g   Carbs: 15g   Protein: 24g

The Total Protein intake is 67.3 grams of protein. I would have 1 scoop of protein - 25grams - after your workout making a grand total of 92.3.

Notice how the carbs are minimal - except after your training. You can have carbs then, then stick with veg and fruit.

Tuesday - Cardio

<u>Before Breakfast:</u>

Do 10 minutes of stretches and then go for an early half hour run - outside or use the running machine in a gym.

Be sure to warm down, and remember that you are walking today - do as much as you can.

Nutrition

Upon Waking:

Have a long glass of warm water with lemon - either fresh lemon or pure lemon dripped in.

12 P.M - Breakfast - Meal One

- 1 x multivitamin
- 1 x Whey Protein shake - with peanut butter and a banana
- 1 30gram x Bowl of Granola

NUTRITION FACTS

Calories: 561   Fat: 30.4 g   Carbs: 26.2 g   Protein: 28 g

4 P.M - Lunch - Meal Two

- 1 x Medium sized Tuna Steak
- 1 x Cup Vegetables/salad

NUTRITION FACTS

Calories: 471   Fat: 33.2 g   Carbs: 17 g   Protein: 27 g

7 PM - Dinner - Meal Three

- Tuna Steak
- Rocket and sliced Red Peppers
- Medium Sweet Potato

NUTRITION FACTS

Calories: 456   Fat: 17g Carbs: 29g   Protein: 28g

The Total Protein intake is 83 grams of protein. I would have 1 scoops of protein plus after your workout making a grand total of 108.

Wednesday - Cardio

<u>**Cardio**</u>

Do this 3 times. Go!

Three circuits: 10 reps per exercise. No rests.

Round One:

- **Burpees**
- **Press-ups**
- **Jumping Jacks**

- **Skipping rope: 3 minutes**

Rest 1 minute

Three circuits: 20 reps per exercise. No rest

Round Two:

- **Walking Lunges with kettlebell exchange underneath leg**
- **Star jumps**
- **High knees running on the spot**

- **Skipping rope: 5 minutes**

Rest 1 minute

Three circuits: 30 reps per exercise. No rest.

Round Three:

- **Pullups**
- **Box Jumps**
- **Star jumps**

- **Skipping rope: 5 minutes**

Rest 1 minute

Three circuits: 40 reps per move. No Rest

Round Four:

- **Alternate Side Lunges**
- **Dips**
- **Shadow boxing**

Nutrition

Upon Waking:

Have a long glass of warm water with lemon - either fresh lemon or pure lemon dripped in.

12 P.M - Breakfast - Meal One

- 1 x multivitamin
- 2 boiled eggs
- Porridge Oats 30gram serving with 1 tbsp. honey

NUTRITION FACTS

Calories: 409   Fat: 17.6 g   Carbs: 35.6 g   Protein: 20.3 g

4 P.M - Lunch - Meal Two

- Full-Fat Cottage Cheese
- 1 cup Cashews
- 1 Pear
- 1 Banana

NUTRITION FACTS

Calories: 566   Fat: 17 g   Carb: 59 g   Protein: 28 g

7 P.M - Dinner - Meal Three

- Pork Chops 5 ounces- with cooked apple - cooked together
- Vegetables 1 cup

NUTRITION FACTS

Calories: 380   Fat: 18.2 g   Carbs: 25 g   Protein: 28 g

The Total Protein intake is 76.3 grams of protein. I would have
1 scoop of protein after your workout making a grand total of
101.3.

Thursday - Cardio

Before Breakfast:

Do 10 minutes of stretches and then go for an early half hour of spinning or a bike ride - outside or use the running machine in a gym.

Or just stick to the pavement and do a 40-minute run. Remember to warm down.

Nutrition

Upon Waking:

Have a long glass of warm water with lemon - either fresh lemon or pure lemon dripped in.

12 P.M - Breakfast - Meal One

- 1 x multivitamin
- 1 x Whey Protein shake - with peanut butter and a banana
- 1 30gram x Bowl of Granola

NUTRITION FACTS

Calories: 561   Fat: 30.4 g   Carbs: 26.2 g   Protein: 28 g

4 P.M Lunch - Meal Two

- 1 x can of Tuna Steak
- Rocket and Beetroot

NUTRITION FACTS

Calories: 471   Fat: 33.2 g   Carbs: 17 g   Protein: 27 g

7 P.M Dinner - Meal Three

- Chicken Breast - With parsley, and bell peppers sliced up
- Steamed Broccoli

NUTRITION FACTS

Calories: 318   Fat: 15g   Carbs: 15g   Protein: 24g

The Total Protein intake is 79 grams of protein. I would have 1 scoops of protein plus after your workout making a grand total of 104.

Friday - Cardio

Cardio

Do this 3 times. Go!

Three circuits: 10 reps per exercise. No rests.

Round One:

- **Burpees**
- **Press-ups**
- **Jumping Jacks**

- **Skipping rope: 5 minutes**

Rest 1 minute

Three circuits: 20 reps per exercise. No rest

Round Two:

- **Walking Lunges with kettlebell exchange underneath leg**
- **Star jumps**
- **High knees running on the spot**

- **Skipping rope: 5 minutes**

Rest 1 minute

Three circuits: 30 reps per exercise. No rest.

Round Three:

- **Pullups**
- **Box Jumps**
- **Star jumps**

- **Skipping rope: 5 minutes**

Rest 1 minute

Three circuits: 40 reps per move. No Rest

Round Four:

- **Alternate Side Lunges**
- **Dips**
- **Shadow boxing**

Nutrition

Upon Waking:

Have a long glass of warm water with lemon - either fresh lemon or pure lemon dripped in.

12 P.M - Breakfast - Meal One

- 1 x multivitamin
- 2 Whole Eggs Scrambled
- Mixed with Green beans cut up

NUTRITION FACTS

Calories: 409   Fat: 17.6 g   Carbs: 20.6 g   Protein: 16.3 g

4 P.M Lunch - Meal Two

- 1 x Medium sized Tuna Steak
- 1 x Cup Vegetables/salad
- 1 Medium sized Baked Potato

NUTRITION FACTS

Calories: 571   Fat: 33.2 g   Carbs: 80 g   Protein: 33 g

7 P.M - Dinner - Meal Three

- Chicken Breast - With parsley, and bell peppers sliced up
- Sprouts - cooked and mashed - add pepper and soft cheese - mash up

NUTRITION FACTS

Calories: 418   Fat: 15g   Carbs: 28g   Protein: 29g

The Total Protein intake is 78.3 grams of protein. I would have 1 scoop of protein - 25grams - after your workout making a grand total of 103.3.

Saturday - Cardio

Before Breakfast

1.5 hours of swimming or 1 x 50-minute insanity workout or 2 30 minute runs.

Remember to warm up before and cool down after.

Nutrition

Upon Waking:

Have a long glass of warm water with lemon - either fresh lemon or pure lemon dripped in.

12 P.M - Breakfast - Meal One

- 1 x multivitamin
- 2 boiled eggs
- Porridge Oats 30gram serving with 1 tbsp. honey

NUTRITION FACTS

Calories: 409   Fat: 17.6 g   Carbs: 35.6 g   Protein: 20.3 g

4 P.M - Lunch - Meal Two

- Full-Fat Cottage Cheese
- 1 cups Cashews
- 1 Apple

NUTRITION FACTS

Calories: 356   Fat: 17 g   Carb: 9 g   Protein: 26 g

7 P.M - Dinner - Meal Three

- Pork Chops 5 ounces- with cooked apple - cooked together
- Vegetables 1 cup

NUTRITION FACTS

Calories: 380   Fat: 18.2 g   Carbs: 25 g   Protein: 28 g

The Total Protein intake is 74.3 grams of protein. I would have 1 scoop of protein after your workout making a grand total of 99.3.

Sunday - Rest and Nutrition

We're one week away from the end of our workout! As per usual, relax and enjoy your cheat meal.

Upon Waking:

Have a long glass of warm water with lemon - either fresh lemon or pure lemon dripped in.

Breakfast - Meal One

- 1 x multivitamin
- 3 x scrambled eggs - with spinach
- 1 30gram x Bowl of Granola

NUTRITION FACTS

Calories: 561   Fat: 30.4 g   Carbs: 26.2 g   Protein: 26 g

Lunch - Meal Two

CHEAT MEAL - whatever you fancy!

7 P.M - Dinner - Meal Three

- 1 Cup x Full-Fat Cottage Cheese
- 1 x blob of peanut butter mixed in

NUTRITION FACTS

Calories: 371   Fat: 27 g   Carb: 9 g   Protein: 24 g

15. Week 10 Workout Yoga

Finally, it's the last week. You've worked so hard and I'm proud you have made it this far. Let's make this final week count!

Monday

Warm-up, or meditate, by sitting cross-legged on the floor. Do this after your wake-up water but before breakfast.

Yoga

I have already explained the yoga positions from week 3, so they all apply. For week 6, you're going to try and reach further and hold the positions longer.

Cow and Cat pose – Switch 10 times.
Downward Dog pose – Rise and fall. Repeat 10 times.
Extended Side Angle – Start left leg, then right. Hold for 6 breathers each.

Child's Pose – Hold for 10 breathers.

Rest break of 1 minute

Downward Dog pose – Repeat 10 times

Extended Side Angle – Start left, then right. Hold for 6 breathers each.
Cow and Cat pose – Switch 10 times

Child Pose – Hold for 10 breathers.

Rest for 5 minutes, end session.

Nutrition

<u>Upon Waking:</u>

Have a long glass of warm water with lemon - either fresh lemon or pure lemon dripped in.

<u>12 PM Breakfast – Meal One</u>

- 1 x multivitamin
- An Orange
- Mixed with Green beans cut up

NUTRITION FACTS

Calories: 289   Fat: 4.4 g   Carbs: 34 g   Protein: 5.3 g

<u>4 PM Lunch – Meal Two</u>

- Fruit Salad Cup (Peach, Pear, Apricot, Pineapple, Cherry)
- Frozen Yogurt

NUTRITION FACTS
Calories: 275 Fat: 2.1g Carbs: 49.5g Protein: 21.3g

<u>7 PM Dinner – Meal Three</u>

- Smooth Peanut-Butter Sandwich (2 cups, 2 slices of bread)
- Apple

NUTRITION FACTS

Calories: 442 Fat: 18.3g Carbs: 60.3g Protein: 15.8

Total protein gain is 42.4 g. Again, no protein cups for yoga week.

Tuesday

Meditate cross-legged style for 15 breaths. Do this after the wake-up water but before breakfast.

<u>Yoga</u>

Mountain Pose – 6 breathers, reach higher each time.

Tree Pose – 25 breathers for each leg.
Warrior Pose – 25 breathers for each leg.

Pidgeon Pose – 25 breathers for each leg.

Rest for 1 minute.

Pidgeon Pose – 25 breathers for each leg.

Tree Pose – 25 breathers for each leg.

Mountain Pose – 6 breathers, reach higher each time
Warrior Pose – 25 breathers for each leg.

Rest for 5 minutes, end session.

Nutrition

Upon Waking:

Have a long glass of warm water with lemon - either fresh lemon or pure lemon dripped in.

12 PM Breakfast – Meal One

- 1 x multivitamin
- An Orange
- Mixed with Green beans cut up

NUTRITION FACTS

Calories: 289   Fat: 4.4 g   Carbs: 34 g   Protein: 5.3 g

4 PM Lunch – Meal Two

- Fruit Salad Cup (Peach, Pear, Apricot, Pineapple, Cherry)
- Frozen Yogurt

NUTRITION FACTS
Calories: 275 Fat: 2.1g Carbs: 49.5g Protein: 21.3g

7 PM Dinner – Meal Three

- Smooth Peanut-Butter Sandwich (2 cups, 2 slices of bread)

- Apple

NUTRITION FACTS

Calories: 442 Fat: 18.3g Carbs: 60.3g Protein: 15.8

Total protein gain is 42.4 g.

Wednesday

Meditate cross-legged style for 15 breaths. Do this after wake-up water but before breakfast.

<u>Yoga</u>

Bridge Pose –Hold for 25 breathers.

Cobra Pose – Rise and fall 10 times.

Crow Pose – Hold for 15 breathers.

Seated Twist – 25 breathers for each side.

Rest for 1 minute.

Seated Twist – 25 breathers for each side.

Cobra Pose – Rise and fall 10 times.

Bridge Pose – Hold for 25 breathers.

Crow Pose – Hold for 15 breathers

Nutrition

Upon Waking:

Have a long glass of warm water with lemon - either fresh lemon or pure lemon dripped in.

12 PM Breakfast – Meal One

- 1 x multivitamin
- An Orange
- Porridge Oats 30gram serving with 1 tbsp. honey

NUTRITION FACTS

Calories: 427 Fat: 8.2g   Carbs: 50.2g Protein: 8.9 g

4 P.M - Lunch - Meal Two

- Full-Fat Cottage Cheese
- 1 cups Cashews
- 1 Apple

NUTRITION FACTS

Calories: 356   Fat: 17 g Carb: 9 g   Protein: 26 g

7 PM Dinner – Meal Three

- Canned Tomato Soup
- Full-Fat Cottage Cheese
- Saltine Crackers

NUTRITION FACTS

Calories: 292 Fat: 7.2g Carb: 41g Protein: 18.7g

Total protein gain is 53.6g. Remember not to eat any protein cups this week.

Thursday

Meditate cross-legged style for 15 breaths. Do this after wake-up water but before breakfast.

<u>Yoga</u>

Again, flow and hold the positions for three breaths for each. Once you are done, switch back to the warm-up cross-leg position to rest.

Cow and Cat pose – Switch from Cow to Cat 10 times.
Downward Dog pose – Hold and then switch 10 times
Extended Side Angle – switch legs after 7 breathers
Child's Pose – hold for 10 breaths

Rest break of 1 minute

Downward Dog pose – repeat 10 times

Extended Side Angle – switch legs after 7 breathers
Cow and Cat pose – switch 10 times

Child Pose – hold for 10 breathers.

Rest for 5 minutes, end session.

Nutrition

Upon Waking:

Have a long glass of warm water with lemon - either fresh lemon or pure lemon dripped in.

12 PM Breakfast – Meal One

- 1 x multivitamin
- An Orange
- Mixed with Green beans cut up

NUTRITION FACTS

Calories: 289   Fat: 4.4 g   Carbs: 34 g   Protein: 5.3 g

4 PM Lunch – Meal Two

- Fruit Salad Cup (Peach, Pear, Apricot, Pineapple, Cherry)
- Frozen Yogurt

NUTRITION FACTS
Calories: 275 Fat: 2.1g Carbs: 49.5g Protein: 21.3g

7 PM Dinner – Meal Three

- Smooth Peanut-Butter Sandwich (2 cups, 2 slices of bread)
- Apple

NUTRITION FACTS

Calories: 442 Fat: 18.3g Carbs: 60.3g Protein: 15.8

Total protein gain is 42.4g.

Friday

Meditate cross-legged style for 15 breaths. Do this after wake-up water but before breakfast.

Seated Twist – 25 breathers for each side.
Pidgeon Pose – 25 breathers per leg.
Downward Dog – repeat 10 times.
Child Pose – hold for 10 breathers.

Rest for 1 minute.

Pidgeon Pose – 25 breathers per leg.
Downward Dog – repeat 10 times.
Seated Twist – 25 breathers for each side.

Child Pose – hold for 10 breathers.

Rest for 5 minutes. End session.

Nutrition

Upon Waking:

Have a long glass of warm water with lemon - either fresh lemon or pure lemon dripped in.

12 PM Breakfast – Meal One

- 1 x multivitamin
- An Orange
- Porridge Oats 30gram serving with 1 tbsp. honey

NUTRITION FACTS

Calories: 427 Fat: 8.2 g   Carbs: 50.2g Protein: 8.9 g

4 PM Lunch – Meal Two

- Full-Fat Cottage Cheese
- 1 cups Cashews
- 1 Apple

NUTRITION FACTS

Calories: 356   Fat: 17 g Carb: 9 g   Protein: 26 g

7 PM Dinner – Meal Three

- Smooth Peanut-Butter Sandwich (2 cups, 2 slices of bread)
- Apple

NUTRITION FACTS

Calories: 442 Fat: 18.3g Carbs: 60.3g Protein: 15.8

Total protein gain is 50.7g

Saturday

Tree Pose – 15 breathers for each leg.

Extended Side Angle – switch legs between 3 breathers
Mountain Pose – 3 breathers, reach higher each time

Warrior Pose – 15 breathers for each leg.

Rest for 1 minute.

Mountain Pose – 3 breathers, reach higher each time.
Warrior Pose – 15 breathers for each leg.

Extended Side Angle – switch legs between 3 breathers.

Tree Pose – 15 breathers for each leg

Rest for 5 minutes. End session.

Nutrition

Upon Waking:

Have a long glass of warm water with lemon - either fresh lemon or pure lemon dripped in.

12 P.M - Breakfast - Meal One

- 1 x multivitamin
- An Orange
- Porridge Oats 30gram serving with 1 tbsp. honey

NUTRITION FACTS

Calories: 427 Fat: 8.2g   Carbs: 50.2g Protein: 8.9 g

4 P.M - Lunch - Meal Two

- Full-Fat Cottage Cheese
- 1 cups Cashews
- 1 Apple

NUTRITION FACTS

Calories: 356   Fat: 17 g Carb: 9 g   Protein: 26 g

7 P.M Dinner

- Canned Tomato Soup
- Full-Fat Cottage Cheese
- Saltine Crackers

NUTRITION FACTS

Calories: 292 Fat: 7.2g Carb: 41g Protein: 18.7g

Total protein gain is 53.6g

Sunday - Rest and Nutrition

You did it! You finished all 6 weeks of your Intermittent Fasting diet workout!

By now your body should be strong as an ox, pumped as a dog, and limber as a snake. From here your workout routine should be smooth sailing, whether you want to keep pushing yourself or not. As a reward for your diligence and persistence, you'll get THREE cheat meals this time!

Upon Waking:

Have a long glass of warm water with lemon - either fresh lemon or pure lemon dripped in.

Breakfast - Meal One

CHEAT MEAL – whatever you fancy!

Lunch - Meal Two

CHEAT MEAL - whatever you fancy!

Dinner - Meal

CHEAT MEAL - whatever you fancy!

16. Healthy Foods to Help with Fat loss and Looking Great

Chapter 1: Breakfasts

The thing about the foods you will find in this chapter and others, is that you most likely already eat them. You might not eat them often or you might be eating them every meal. When you eat a well-balanced breakfast, with vegetables, fruit, eggs, oatmeal, and other suggestions found in here, you are getting the antioxidants, anti-inflammatories, and collagen your skin needs to remain healthy. A combination of vitamin C, D, E, A, K, and beta-carotene found in pumpkin, carrots, and other orange fruits lll provide collagen and properties to rejuvenate your skin.

1. Green Eggs and Ham Omelet

Are you a fan of green eggs and ham? Well, we have a new take on the children's favorite that you can incorporate into a delicious, fun and nutrition packed breakfast. The secret to this delightful addition is spinach. The fact is, spinach is one of the best ways to keep you healthy and glowing.

Ingredients:

- 2 eggs

- 1 slice of ham or half cup cubed

- 1 ounce or 1 slice of cheddar cheese

- ½ cup fresh small leaf spinach

- ¼ cup chopped green pepper

Combine all the ingredients into your nutrition blender to mix until blended. The pan should be preheated and sprayed with cooking oil or butter. Cook until done. Serves one.

2. Fruit Salad with Tropical Feel

Antioxidants abound in this "feel the ocean breeze" fruit salad. Not only will your skin reap the benefits of the fresh fruit ingredients, the potassium from cantaloupe and bananas are good for keeping your blood pressure lower. Potassium is also a known ingredient to prevent cramps in your limbs.

Ingredients:

- 1 cup vanilla yogurt, low fat
- 1 teaspoon grated lime zest
- 2 red grapefruits
- 2 kiwi fruit, peeled and cut into small wedges
- 2 bananas, sliced
- 1 small cantaloupe, cut into chunks
- 1 large papaya, seeded and cut into chunks
- 2 tablespoons crystallized ginger

Combine first two ingredients in a small bowl. Prepare the fruits in a large bowl, sectioning the grapefruits over the bowl to catch the juices Squeeze the peels to get all the juice from the membranes. Add the rest of the fruit and ginger. This serves six. Divide the fruit into small bowls and top with the yogurt mixture.

3. Frittata with Zucchini

Zucchini is a rich source of flavonoids, that harm free radicals, which play a role in the aging process. It is low in calories and contain a wonderful bounty of vitamin C another good antioxidant. Add juice or fresh fruit and you have another skin protector against aging.

Ingredients:

- 4 eggs
- 4 egg whites
- ¼ cup of Parmesan cheese
- ¼ teaspoon Mediterranean Sea salt
- 2 tablespoons olive oil
- 1 clove, minced garlic
- 2 small zucchinis, shredded
- 2 red peppers, cut into strips

Eggs provide the protein and using half the yolks ensure that cholesterol levels are kept in check. Preheat the oven to 400 degrees. In a medium bowl, whisk the first four ingredients. Heat oil in a skillet that can be placed in the oven, add garlic and cook for one minute or until just tender. Add the zucchini and peppers and cook for another minute. Pour in the egg mixture and cook about three minutes or until the bottom of the mixture is set. Bake in the oven to finish cooking, about ten minutes.

4. Oatmeal with Berries and Spice

Oatmeal is another staple to have on your pantry shelf. Adding berries, spices, and nuts to the bowl, will add the antioxidants you need for a glowing complexion. The nutrients in this power food support skin health. Add a hardboiled egg for protein and you have a great way to begin your day.

Ingredients:

- ½ cup oatmeal, steel cut, rolled or quick cooking

- ¼ cup berries, blueberries, strawberries, peaches, raspberries, or bananas

- 1/8 teaspoon pumpkin spice

- 1/8 cup chopped nuts, walnuts, pecans, or almonds

Prepare oatmeal according to package directions. If you use steel cut oatmeal you can make a family breakfast in a slow cooker. Wake up to a delicious meal without the fuss. Use 1 cup of oats to 3 cups of water. After the oatmeal is cooked, add the spice, berries and nuts. A sprinkle of brown sugar can be added to taste.

5. Breakfast Sandwich with Kale

If you like a breakfast sandwich you can find a great one for your skin with kale. Don't think traditional breakfast muffin, these delightful gems are cooked in a muffin tin with eggs.

Ingredients:

- Kale

- Half dozen eggs

- Peppers

- Onions

- Mushrooms

- Milk or Coconut Milk

Combine the ingredients into a blender, mix into a smooth consistency, add a tsp milk or coconut milk per egg, whip, and put in a muffin tin. Bake at 350 degrees F for 10 to 15 minutes, or until egg is fully cooked. You can also substitute for other vegetables. Any vegetables mentioned in this chapter that are good for skin glow can be used in your egg muffin.

6. Italian Omelet

The Italian omelet is going to provide eggs, which are healthy for your heart. It also contains tomatoes, which are known to help fight sunburn, reduce skin roughness, and boost collagen.

Ingredients:

- 1 Tbsp. chopped green bell pepper
- 1 Tbsp. chopped onion
- 1 Tbsp. chopped tomatoes + a little extra for garnish
- 2 eggs, beaten
- 1 tsp Italian seasoning
- 1 tsp fresh Parmesan cheese

Place the egg in the pan, after you have beaten them. Once the egg starts to cook add the vegetables.

7. Walnut Pancakes

Adding walnuts to pancakes will help you boost your skin health due to the omega-3 fatty acids, according to Dr. Drayer.

Ingredients:

- 1 cup quick cooking oats
- 3 Tbsp. chopped walnuts
- ½ cup whole grain pastry flour
- 1 ½ tsp baking powder
- 1 tsp ground cinnamon
- 3 egg whites
- 1 tsp pure vanilla
- 1 scoop vanilla whey protein powder
- ½ cup fat free ricotta cheese
- ¾ cup milk

Get your skillet warming, with a little cooking spray or butter. The heat should be on low. Combine the dry ingredients and mix well. Combine the wet ingredients in a separate bowl, then add them to the dry ingredients, mixing well. Let the mix sit for 2 minutes, then start making pancakes.

8. Chocolate Banana Muffins

Research shows dark chocolate has a healthy effect on your skin by offering it hydration and decreasing scaling.

Ingredients:

- 1 ½ cup walnuts
- ¾ cup semisweet dark chocolate baking chips
- 1 ½ cup flour
- 1 Tbsp. baking powder
- ½ cup brown sugar
- ½ tsp cinnamon
- ¼ cup canola oil
- ¼ cup milk
- ¼ cup Greek yogurt (plain)
- 1 egg
- 1 ripe banana, mashed
- 1 tsp vanilla

Preheat the oven to 375 degrees F. Combine the wet ingredients in one bowl and the dry ingredients in the other. Leave the banana out for now. Combine the wet ingredients into the dry, then add the banana as the last step. Put the mix into muffin tins. Cook for 20 minutes in the oven.

9. Bagel with Lox and Cream Cheese

Lox is filled with omega 3-fatty acids, which you know helps your skin.

Ingredients:

- Use fat free cream cheese
- Smoked salmon
- Cucumber, sliced
- Tomato sliced
- Leaves of lettuce
- Choice of bagel

Using a choice of bagel, spread 1 Tbsp. of cream cheese on each side of the bagel. Place 1 to 3 ounces of salmon on the bagel. Top it will lettuce, cucumber, and tomato.

10. Quick Breakfast

Whole grains are full of antioxidants, which help your complexion. Many cereals like Total also have zinc, which is an anti-inflammatory vitamin. Using cereal combined with a banana you can increase your collagen as well as your overall skin health.

Ingredients:

- 1 cup cereal (whole grain such as Total)

- 1 banana, sliced

- Milk

- 2 tsp walnuts, chopped

Simply add each element to a bowl, with enough milk to please your palette and eat.

Chapter 2: Lunches

Your body requires a mixture of various proteins, vitamins, and minerals to be healthy and fight disease. For lunches you want to make certain you are eating a high amount of protein, fewer carbohydrates, and plenty of fruits and vegetables. The recipe suggestions in this section all focus on the main meal, but remember you can always add as many vegetables as you want not only to increase your food intake, but also to ensure your skin continues to glow.

1. Shrimp with Grapefruit

Antioxidant grapefruit again makes an appearance to help your skin glow.

Ingredients:

- 1 red grapefruit
- 1 teaspoon Dijon mustard
- ½ teaspoon Himalayan Pink Salt
- ¼ teaspoon black pepper
- 2 tablespoons olive oil
- 1 large head shredded romaine lettuce or spring mix
- 1 avocado, peeled, pitted and chopped
- 1 pound peeled, deveined and cooked large shrimp

Over a large bowl section, the grapefruit allowing juices to drip into bowl. Squeeze the grapefruit rind over the large bowl to gather all the juice. Put the sections in a smaller bowl. Whisk the mustard, salt and pepper into the large bowl with juice. Whisk in oil. Add the lettuce, avocado, shrimp and grapefruit. Toss the ingredients to coat with the juices. Serves 4

2. Tuna with White Bean Salad

Vitamin rich tomatoes are the key to good skin care in this delicious recipe.

Ingredients:

- 1/3 cup tomato juice
- 3 tablespoons lemon juice
- 2 tablespoons olive oil
- 1 tablespoon fresh basil, chopped or 1 teaspoon dried
- ¼ teaspoon salt
- 1 6-ounce can tuna, drained
- 1 can 15 ounces' white beans, drained and rinsed
- 1 medium cucumber, peeled, seeded and chopped
- ¼ cup pitted Kalamata olives, chopped
- 6 cups of mixed salad greens

In a small bowl, whisk together the first five ingredients. In a medium bowl, toss the next four ingredients with one tablespoon of vinaigrette. Divide the greens among four plates. Top with a quarter of the tuna mixture and drizzle with dressing.

3. Sweet Potato Soup

With more than 30 antioxidant compounds in ginger this sweet potato soup recipe is not only full of flavor but skin benefits as well. It removes toxins, prevents damage caused by free radicals and helps with stimulate proper circulation.

Ingredients:

- 2 tablespoon olive oil

- 2 cloves garlic, minced

- 1 large onion, chopped

- 1 red bell pepper, chopped

- 1 teaspoon ground ginger

- 1 teaspoon allspice

- 4 cups low-sodium chicken or vegetable broth

- 2 large sweet potatoes, peeled and cut into 1 inch chunks

- 1 14-ounce can diced tomatoes

- ½ cup natural peanut butter or almond butter

- 1 16-ounce frozen edamame, shelled

- 5 ounces' baby spinach

Start by warming up the broth in a pan, add in the sliced sweet potatoes. Let the potatoes cook until they are partially soft and add in the rest of the ingredients. The peanut butter will help reduce the amount of broth, making the soup a little thicker.

4. Kale Salad with Pomegranate Seeds and Lemon Vinaigrette

The ingredients in this salad provide plenty of antioxidants, including vitamin K, which are both known to help your skin look younger and fight the aging process. Pomegranate seeds also contain polyphenols, which are in tea, as well, and help with healthy skin and body.

Ingredients:

- Avocado
- Kale
- Quinoa
- Pecans
- Goat Cheese
- Lemon Vinaigrette
- Pomegranate Seeds
- Romaine lettuce
- Spinach

For 1 cup of lettuce, add in as many of the vegetables as you want, use 1 Tbsp. of pecans, 1 ounce of goat cheese, and 2 Tbsp. of the lemon vinaigrette. For the seeds, simply add 1 Tbsp.

5. Lemon Herb Salmon

You have seen salmon before in a breakfast recipe. The same principle applies here for healthier skin.

Ingredients:

- 3 ounces of Salmon
- One lemon
- Ginger
- Garlic
- Celery seeds
- Oregano

Use the herbs to taste. Simply place them over the salmon and squeeze the lemon juice onto the fish. Lay sliced lemon over the salmon, bake it at 350 degrees F until it is cooked. Depending on the thickness of the salmon it may take 10 to 20 minutes.

6. Chicken Salad with Nuts

Chicken is a healthy food, not only because it is low in cholesterol, but because of its antioxidant properties. Combine it with walnuts and cranberries and you will definitely add healthy components that help your skin.

Ingredients:

- 2 Tbsp. mayo
- ½ pound chicken
- Whole grain bread
- ¼ cup cranberries
- ¼ cup walnuts

Combine the ingredients in a bowl, with the chicken, diced, then spread the chicken salad over the bread.

7. Chicken Pot Pie

Chicken pot pie allows you to get vegetables, meat, potatoes, and crust all in one. The vegetables you use can all lend a hand in keeping your skin glowing and fight aging; especially if you combine spinach, kale, or tomatoes into your pie.

Ingredients:

- Celery

- Tomatoes

- Potatoes

- Carrots

- Chicken

- Pie crust

- Chicken Gravy

This lunch will need to be made the night before. Heat the oven to 350 degrees F. Place a crust in the bottom of a pie pan. Dice your chicken and vegetables. Put them in the pie pan in a nice even layer. Layer the ingredients with the gravy, place the second crust on the top and bake for 30 minutes. If you do not like tomatoes, spinach or kale in the pie, you can have that as your side dish such as a spinach salad.

8. Broccoli Chicken Stir-fry

Stir-fry is just a way to say you have a lot of vegetables and meat to place over Ramen or Rice. What you put in a stir fry is up to you, but if you want healthy skin, then the suggestions for this recipe will definitely provide antioxidants for your skin health, plus vitamins C, E, and A. Broccoli is also known to help with skin regeneration and repair due to a property called glucoraphanin.

Ingredients:

- 1 pound of chicken

- 2 heads of broccoli

- 1 carrot

- 1 cup of seaweed

- Peppers

- Onion

- Water chestnuts

- Bamboo shoots

- If there are any vegetables such as mushrooms that you like, you can add them. The main point is to have the broccoli and chicken in the dish. You can decide to use soy sauce or another stir-fry sauce. One with ginger is a good option since ginger also has antioxidant and anti-inflammatory properties. Brown rice is best for health reasons. Simply cook the chicken, add the carrots and other hard vegetables once the chicken is cooked. Add in the sauce and the rest of the vegetables, let cook until the vegetables are cooked and serve over rice or noodles.

9. Light Lunch Dip

Sometimes you might not want a lot for lunch, but you want it to help you keep your skin healthy. An Edamame Ginger dip can be the light lunch that you want, which is filled with antioxidants and ingredients that will keep you full.

Ingredients:

- Edamame
- 1tbsp Ginger
- 2tbsp Soy Sauce
- ¼ cup water
- 1 tbsp. rice vinegar
- 1 tbsp. tahini
- 1 clove garlic

Cook the edamame until it is soft. Usually you have to buy a frozen shelled edamame, so the instructions are on the package. Puree the edamame with the rest of the ingredients, chill it, and then serve with crackers or carrots. It can also be a dip you have as a side with chicken.

10. Tofu Peanut Wrap

Tofu is considered a healthy alternative to meat. Adding peanuts with red bell pepper and snow peas, also adds antioxidants to the meal.

Ingredients:

- Whole wheat tortilla

- 2 thinly sliced ounces of tofu

- ¼ cup sliced bell pepper

- 8 sliced snow peas

- 1 tbsp. peanut sauce

- 1 tbsp. peanuts

Spread the peanut sauce on the tortilla. Place the other ingredients over the top and fold the tortilla to your preferences.

Chapter 3: Dinners

Many of these dinners are going to contain the same vegetables, chicken, fish and tofu of the lunch recipes. The difference will be in the type of recipe to ensure you have 10 different dinner options. Keep in mind that you can do a lot with the same types of ingredients, with only minor changes to make it more Asian, American, or European.

1. Chicken Fajitas

Chicken Fajitas can be made with your health in mind. Adding vegetables, light cheese, and whole grain tortilla shells to the meal will help you keep your skin healthy.

Ingredients:

- 1 lb. chicken

- 1 green bell pepper

- 1 yellow bell pepper

- 1 red bell pepper

- 1 onion

- Fresh herbs based on your taste

- Garlic

- 1 tbsp. butter

- Whole grain tortilla

Cook the chicken in a skillet with the butter, garlic, and herbs. Add the cut up vegetables, until they are the desired doneness. Put the tortilla in another skillet to warm it up for 30 seconds. Sprinkle some cheese onto the tortilla and add in the chicken mixture. Use Pico de Gallo or Salsa as a garnish to get health benefits from tomatoes.

2. Halibut with Spinach Salad

Halibut is a white fish found on the bottom of the ocean, in cooler temperatures. It is one of the best fish to eat, if you are not a fish fan. While it is not among the highest rated fish for minerals and antioxidants, it still contains omega 3-fatty acids.

Ingredients:

- 3 oz. Halibut

- 1 lemon

- 1 tbsp. butter

- Garlic

- Spinach

- Lemon vinaigrette

- Cranberries

- Walnuts

For the halibut, you can either grill or bake it. For grilling, put the halibut on tin foil. Butter both sides, squeeze lemon on both sides, and place garlic on both sides. Wrap the tin foil and cook for 10 minutes, flip the fish and cook another 5 minutes with the tin foil open. The length of time you cook the fish may vary based on the thickness of the fish. You may need to cook the fish for less time.

In a bowl, combine spinach, romaine if you wish, cranberries, walnuts, and lemon vinaigrette.

3. Homemade Stew

Stew is not only a simple meal, but also one that offers you plenty of different vegetables. The great part about stew is that it was originally made based off of what you had in the house. This means adding in anything you want and it can be called a stew. To make this recipe healthier for your skin, some additions have been added that might not be in your typical recipe.

Ingredients:

- Beef
- Lentils (your choice)
- Brown gravy
- Potatoes
- Leaks
- Carrots
- Celery
- onion
- Kale or spinach
- Tomatoes

For the stew, start it in the morning in your crockpot. Mix up brown gravy from a powder or use beef broth. Add the stew meat, vegetables, beans, and onion. Leave the tomatoes out. The tomatoes will be for later on when you are ready to eat your stew. Let the ingredients mix, cook, and become flavorful throughout the day.

When you are ready to eat, cut up the tomatoes into slices. Using a little salt and pepper to taste, cover the tomatoes. You can eat them raw or if you like you can fry them. You would get the best results out of the raw tomato.

4. Veggie Delight

Vegetables are some of the best foods anyone can eat for a healthy glow. If you are a vegetarian or just tired of meat, you can create a veggie meal.

Ingredients:

- 1 small yellow onion, chopped

- 2 tbsp. butter

- 3 garlic gloves, crushed

- 2 large Portobello mushrooms, sliced

- 2 ½ cups button, brown or cremini mushrooms, sliced

- 1 tbsp. flour

- ½ cup cooked brown lentils, follow the package instructions

- 2 ½ cups vegetable stock

- 1 cup pearl onions, peeled

- 1 pinch of pepper and salt to taste

In a skillet, add the butter, onions, garlic, and mushrooms. Cook until the mushrooms become soft and slightly browned. Add in the lentils and cook for an additional 2 minutes. Sprinkle the flour over the mixture, stir it in, and then add the vegetable stock. Simmer the mixture for 10 minutes or until the sauce becomes thick.

5. Cashew Chicken

Cashew chicken is a favourite among Asian cultures because it provides two types of protein, plus ingredients for a healthy skin and body. Cashews are particularly helpful in the antioxidant department.

- 1 lb. of chicken, sliced
- ½ cup of cashews
- ¼ cup soy sauce
- 1/8 cup peanut sauce
- Wheat noodles
- Vegetables
- Sesame oil

Start by heating up your wok or skillet to 300 degrees or low/medium heat. Pour 1 tbsp. of sesame oil into the pan or use butter if you don't have any. Cook the chicken first. Wait until it is cooked through before adding your choice of vegetables. Any green veggies, such as broccoli, seaweed, or veggies like carrots should be used. Onions and bell peppers are also filled with appropriate nutrients for skin health. Cook the veggies until they are soft. You can also add in the soy sauce and peanut sauce to help steam the veggies. Cook the noodles per package instructions. Once all is cooked, add in the cashews, mix it up and serve.

6. Homemade Spaghetti

Homemade spaghetti sauce is a great way to ensure you have the appropriate vitamins and antioxidants from the tomatoes in your meal.

Ingredients:

- 1 cup water

- A dozen whole tomatoes

- Garlic

- Oregano

- Other herbs

- Using Italian herbs, including oregano and garlic you will season your tomatoes. The choice of herbs is up to you and what you like. Many herbs, including oregano, garlic, and parsley have antioxidants. First, you will need to boil your tomatoes in the water. Using 6 of the tomatoes, boil them until they are soft. The other six tomatoes will be pureed in a blender until a paste starts to form. Add the pureed tomatoes to the tomatoes. This will thicken the sauce. Add in the herbs and let it cook until you have a nice flavor. For the spaghetti, simply choose a whole grain noodle, cook as you normally would.

7. Chicken Lettuce Wraps

Anytime you combine green vegetables like lettuce with chicken you are helping your skin. Lettuce wraps are another Asian dish, which are already known to have health benefits beyond just skin.

Ingredients:

- 1 lb. chicken, cut into strips

- 1 cup of water

- 1 package of lettuce wrap seasoning

- 1 bell pepper

- 1 carrot

- Green onions

- Romaine lettuce

In a skillet or wok, cook the chicken. You can use butter or sesame oil to ensure the chicken does not stick to the pan. Add the seasoning and water after the chicken is cooked, along with the vegetables, save the lettuce. While the chicken is cooking, clean the Romaine lettuce, lay out entire leaves, and then put the cooked chicken concoction in a bowl. Simply put a spoonful of chicken into the lettuce and eat it. If you would like, you can use a food processor to reduce the chicken in size for an easier time eating it.

8. Pork with Apricot Sauce

Apricots are very healthy for your skin; they can also make a great addition to pork. You will want to use a lean pork roast or pork chop to keep the cholesterol down.

Ingredients:

- 1 lb. pork
- ¼ cup Dijon
- ¼ cup apricot jelly or fresh apricots
- 1 onion
- ½ cup vegetable or chicken broth

In a skillet, put the vegetable broth, and onion in and place the pork into the pan. Cook one side. After you turn the pork over, dump the Dijon mustard and apricot mixture into the skillet. If you use fresh apricots, they need to be cut into chunks and the juice squeezed into the pan. Cook until the other side of the pork is nicely cooked. It takes about 20 minutes. Serve with the sauce to help keep the pork moist.

9. Chicken and Mandarin Salad

Green vegetables, orange fruits, and chicken make a nice compliment for a light dinner.

Ingredients:

- Romaine lettuce
- Spinach
- Mandarin oranges
- Apricots
- Apples
- 1 chicken breast or 2 tenderloins
- Salad toppings of choice

For this recipe it is about combining fruit, lettuce, and chicken, so you have a complete meal all in one bowl. It is up to you whether you use croutons, wontons, fried onions, or chow mien noodles in your salads. You also want to choose a low fat dressing or vinaigrette. You can also add more fruits and vegetables like peppers, broccoli, cranberries and blueberries to the salad.

10. Spaghetti Pie

Spaghetti Pie is a casserole dish you can create. It takes a little prep, sometime in the oven, and then you have a meal you can eat quickly. The tomatoes will bring the healthy skin glow you are looking for.

Ingredients:

- Whole grain spaghetti

- Tomato sauce, preferably homemade

- Light or fat free ricotta

- Hamburger

- Mozzarella

Cook the spaghetti noodles as you would normally do. Cook the hamburger, drain the oil and fat, then combine with the sauce. You don't have to heat the sauce. Instead, you will mix the ricotta into the sauce and pour it over the hot spaghetti, mix in the noodles, put mozzarella over the top and bake it. You will need to heat the oven to 350 degrees F, put the ingredients in a pie pan, and cook for 25 to 30 minutes.

Chapter 4: Snacks

Snacks can be just as healthy, whether you eat them throughout the day or at night. You definitely need to combine plenty of vegetables and fruits in your snacks to ensure you are eating healthy. Nuts, fruits, and vegetables all contain antioxidants, anti-inflammatory, and polyphenols that help your skin glow, rejuvenate, and lose its scaly appearance. The snacks in this section will contain these properties to ensure you have a healthy glow.

1. Blueberry Fruit Salad

Blueberries are one of the highest fruits when it comes to antioxidants and skin care. Creating a fruit salad around blueberries is simple, quick, and extremely healthy.

Ingredients:

- Blueberries
- Strawberries
- Bananas
- Kiwi
- Apricots

The main ingredient should be blueberries, but really all you need to do is slice the various other fruits, put them in a bowl and decide if you wish to add a little yogurt for protein.

2. Strawberries and Cream

For this recipe, you are taking healthy strawberries and adding them to Greek yogurt. Your other options are to use heavy whip, mix it in a mixing bowl, and dip your strawberries for a little dessert. It can also be substituted with any other fruit, including oranges, apricots, pineapple, and blueberries.

3. Artichoke Dip

Artichokes are good for your health and your skin. Like many vegetables they contain powerful properties such as anti-inflammatory and antioxidants.

Ingredients:

- 1 can artichoke hearts or fresh artichoke

- 1 cup mayo

- 1 cup grated, fresh Parmesan cheese

Preheat the oven to 375 degrees F. Combine the artichoke hearts with the other two ingredients, blend in a blender to mix well and break the hearts up a little bit. Spread into a 9x13 inch pan, bake for 15 to 20 minutes and then serve warm or cold. Serve with whole grain bread or crackers.

4. Spinach Dip

Spinach is that lovely green vegetable that you should eat more of given its healthful properties, some of which have already been discussed. Like the anti-inflammatory properties of most vegetables, you also find this in spinach.

Ingredients:

- 1 cup mayo

- 1 package of leek soup mix

- 1 16-oz sour cream

- 1 4-oz can water chestnuts, finely chopped

- 10 ounces of spinach

Mix the ingredients in a bowl. Refrigerator for 6 hours and then serve. You can serve with whole grain crackers or bread.

5. Salsa and Whole Grain Chips

Making your own salsa ensures it has everything you want in it. Tomatoes, as many of the recipes have been saying are good for skin based on the antioxidants they have.

Ingredients:

- Tomatoes
- Peppers
- Onions
- Jalapenos
- Tomato juice

Dice up the tomatoes and other vegetables as small as you wish. You can leave it as a chunky salsa or even use a food processor to reduce the size of the vegetables. Use the tomato juice from the tomatoes to mix the salsa. The amount of peppers and jalapenos will determine how spicy the food is. For every tomato you use, add the same amount as the other vegetables. The chips should be a whole grain choice.

6. Yellow and Orange Fruit Salad

Fruit salads can truly be made with anything you wish. If you are looking for more of a dessert than a fruit bowl, consider the following fruits combined with cream cheese and sweetened condensed milk.

Ingredients:

- 1 8-ounce cream cheese
- ½ can sweetened condensed milk
- 1 can mandarin oranges
- 1 orange
- ½ cup pineapple
- 1 peach
- 1 banana

Any yellow and orange fruit will be rich in antioxidants and help promote skin health. You can leave out some of the fruit or add in more. Let the cream cheese reach room temperature, so you can whip it. Add the condensed milk to make a nice, slightly runny mixture and then add all the fruit.

7. Carrots, Broccoli, and Dip

While not strictly a recipe, getting a vegetable platter with carrots, broccoli, radishes, peppers, and celery can make a nice snack. You can also create your own platter from home grown vegetables. The dip should be homemade too, for better quality.

You can use spinach or artichoke dip or the following:

- 1 cup sour cream

- 1 package ranch mix or herbs you grow

Combine the ingredients, let it sit in the fridge for an hour and serve.

8. Homemade Trail Mix

Trail mix by definition is full of nuts and fruits. There is nothing better than making your own trail mix. You can even put a few dark chocolate pieces in to help with your skin care.

- ½ cup raisins

- ½ cup walnuts

- ½ cup pecans

- ½ cup cashews

- ½ cup dried fruits (choose bananas, blueberries, cranberries, or any fruits)

- ½ cup dark chocolate pieces

Take all the ingredients, put them in a bag, shake it up, and eat it whenever you feel hungry.

9. Tuna Finger Sandwiches

Tuna is one of the best fish to make into a sandwich for a snack. You can make little finger sandwiches to serve on whole grain bread when you host a party, tea, or simply when you want a snack for the whole family.

- 1 package of Tuna

- 2 tbsp mayo, light or fat free

- Whole grain bread

Cut the bread with cookie cutters, making sure to also cut the crust off. Mix the tuna and mayo, spread it on the bread and serve. You can also add pits of celery if you prefer. Another option is to top the top piece of bread with a small green, yellow, or red pepper. It gives you another boost of antioxidants.

10. Cucumber Sandwiches and Slices

The great thing about cucumber is its anti-inflammatory properties. You can put slices on your eyes, let it help with the bags you have, and then eat the cucumber that is leftover to get even more antioxidants and anti-inflammatory properties.

For the recipe:

Ingredients:

- 1 cucumber

- Cream cheese

- Whole grain bread

- Salt and pepper

To make the sandwiches, use a cookie cutter to get little finger sandwich sizes and cut the crust off. Then spread a thin layer of cream cheese on the bread. This will hold the cucumber in place. You can add salt and pepper to enhance the taste or a little paprika. If you do not want to make a sandwich, simply salt and pepper the cucumber and eat the slices.

Chapter 5: Smoothies

Smoothies are a great way to replace a meal or snack. The right smoothie might have 300 calories with plenty of green vegetables to ensure your healthy skin will continue as you age. The smoothies in this chapter will examine various options from green smoothies to super food smoothies that will definitely contain the antioxidants, anti-inflammatory, and collagen you need to look great.

1. A Very Green Smoothie

If you want to be healthy; especially, to increase the health of your skin, then consider this green smoothie. It doesn't have a great taste, but it will rejuvenate your skin.

Ingredients:

- 1 cup spinach
- 1 small cucumber
- ½ avocado
- 1 leaf from collard greens
- 1 ½ cup water
- 1 leaf from black kale
- ¼ granny smith apple
- 2 lemons

Mix it all in a blender. Add almond or coconut milk to reduce the acidity.

2. Aloe and Apple Delight

Aloe has always been known as the healing plant. Topically, it can help heal cuts faster, as well as prevent scars. Drinking it in a smoothie also helps some of the properties reach your internal cells, particularly to help regenerate new skin cells.

Ingredients:

- 4 collard leaves
- 2 large spears of Aloe, fresh from a plant
- 1-inch fresh ginger, peeled
- 1 banana
- 1 granny smith apple
- 1 ¾ cup ice
- 1 ½ cup blueberries, fresh

Mix everything in the blender. Serve or keep for 24 hours. Adding honey for a little sweetener can also help your skin.

3. Seaweed Asian Smoothie

Seaweed like nori, wakame, and arame are known to contain antioxidants and nutrients that are helpful for the skin as well as your heart. This smoothie can help prevent certain diseases as it lowers cholesterol and adds anti-inflammatory properties to your body.

Ingredients:

- 2 handfuls of arugula
- 1 handful of spinach
- ¼ cup seaweed
- 2 cups pineapple, fresh
- 2 bananas, fresh
- 1 apple
- 3 cups ice
- 2 cups blueberries, fresh

Mix everything in a blender. It makes 3 servings and can be kept for 24 hours.

4. Asian Vegetable Smoothie with Fruit

Bok choy is known for its antioxidants and healthy properties to ensure heart health and prevention of certain diseases. In a smoothie with vegetables and fruits it can also help with your skin.

Ingredients:

- 1 cup Chinese celery

- 8 cups Bok choy, chopped

- 1 cup bean sprouts

- 4 tangelos

- 4 cups mixed berries, fresh

- 2 bananas, fresh

Mix it all in a blender with 2 ¼ cups ice. It will serve 6 people or can be kept for 24 hours.

5. Fruit and Cabbage Smoothie

This smoothie combines the properties of cabbage with fruit to help enhance your skin.

Ingredients:

- 2 cups berries or other fruit
- 1 banana
- ½ green cabbage
- 1 granny smith apple
- 1 ¾ cups ice
- ¼ cup raw agave

Put everything in the blender and mix until smooth.

6. Green Tea Fruit Smoothie

Green tea or any tea has antioxidants and anti-inflammatory properties. Mixing a little green tea infused water in with yellow, orange, or green fruits will ensure a great smoothie for your skin.

Ingredients:

- Brew 1 tsp. green tea and let it cool

- Grab whatever fruits you love in the colour categories named

- Coconut milk

Put ½ a cup of green tea in a blender, add half a dozen ice cubes, and as much fruit choices as you want. Add a tablespoon of coconut milk for the antioxidant properties and protein. Blend well. Use the left over green tea added to flour for a facial mask. You have two skin remedies in one.

7. Tofu and Vegetable Smoothie

You might need to be a hard core vegetarian for this smoothie or like tofu a lot. The vegetables help bring important properties into your body for better skin health. Tofu is great for its protein component.

- 1-ounce tofu

- Spinach and any other green vegetable you like

- Yogurt or coconut milk

In a blender put some ice, the vegetables you like, the tofu, and add enough milk to blend the concoction smooth.

8. Pomegranate, Apple, and Mango Smoothie

All three fruits have the same properties as most fruit, meaning antioxidants, vitamin C and D, which all help healthy skin promotion.

Ingredients:

- 1 fruit (apple, mango, and pomegranate)

- Yogurt, low fat milk or coconut milk

- Ice

De-seed the fruits, put them in a blender, add a cup of milk or yogurt and half a dozen ice cubes. Blend until smooth.

9. Vanilla Kefir and Orange Fruit Smoothie

Vanilla kefir is a drinkable yogurt to add to your smoothie. It has calcium and probiotics to help keep your immune system in check. Add in orange for the vitamin C and D, plus antioxidants for your skin.

Ingredients:

- 2 oranges
- 1 cup vanilla kefir

Blend until smooth in a blender and drink.

10. Whey Protein Vegetable Smoothie

Whey protein for some does not have that great a taste, but it offers you protein in a smoothie, so you can quickly have a well-balanced meal as you move about during your day. The vegetables will enhance your skin health.

Ingredients:

- 1 tbsp. whey protein

- Spinach

- Broccoli

- Kale

- Ice

- ½ cup yogurt

Combine all the ingredients into a blender, mix well, and serve.

17.   CONGRATULATIONS!

Well done for reaching the end of the book! Thank for you purchasing this Book, and congratulations on finishing all 10 weeks!

I hope this book has set you on the road to reaching the fitness you strive for, even if it left your muscles aching. If you deviated or missed the odd day, don't worry, in the scheme of things you have taken steps to improve yourself. In fact in the first few weeks I expect you to take the odd day off. It's tough and is designed that way, especially the last 4 weeks. The important thing is not to overdo it. Learn about your body.

Fitness isn't about one workout or one meal. It's about you committing to the long term to improve yourself. That's all, and by saying I'm going to do this, you have made the first step.

Strive to improve your form for your weights workouts, feel the muscles contract, feel the burn. Make sure you complete your cardio - this is the real fat burner. It is east to skip cardio but trust me, keep on it. Get a partner to help out and follow this with you. Once you string a few sessions of cardio together you'll want to keep it up. I keep checking my pedometer on my phone to see how many steps I've taken as I always strive for more than 6000 every day. So that's around 1 hour of walking. I always park further away than I need too, and I try to walk every morning. This adds to your cardio goals without even trying - so go for it - every little extra counts.

Try to keep to your nutrition. I've put 4pm for your lunch, is this possible for you? If not move it to 5pm or 6:30pm. Make my plan work for you. You are in control and this is a guide that you should use to your advantage. You may need to adjust your nutrition adding more protein, adding more carbs after training if you still feel hungry. You need to get to know how your body responds. If you feel hungry or lethargic increase your healthy food intake a little. You may feel like you're not leaning up, in which case have smaller meals. Reduce your calories.

Keep using the 16 8 Intermittent Fasting routine if you can. Let it last for a month and see how you feel. It won't work wonders in days, it'll take time. And remember it only works when you completely fast for 16 hours - no food at all. Drink plenty of water.

There'll be hard times when you're tired or just want to chill, it's up to you to know when to push on and do that workout or just take a break. Even a 30 minute walk in the evening is better than nothing.

As I said in terms of training you may struggle at first. I would reduce sets - not workouts. Keep to the schedule, keep working the muscles regularly and you will get results.

Number 1 thing to do:

Remember we took a picture at the start? This is really important. We want to see progress. Take a picture before any training, this is what you want to improve upon. Then take a picture every 2 weeks to see how you're progressing. Take a picture at the end of the 10 weeks as well. Then tag me in twitter @usefulebooks

I want to see progress!

Remember

This is fun, it's taking up a portion of your life for the good, so it should never feel like a chore!

Why

Remember why you are doing this. For you, for change, for a healthy life.

Tips

There are a number of cheats I use to maximize muscles gain in terms of supplements.

- A weights Post workout shake is a given - 25grams of Whey Isolate is minimum which will help you recover.
- A scoop of BCAA's in 500ml of water pre-workout and something to sip. Again have this post workout. This is great for recovery and getting you back to feeling normal.

Water

Your body is composed of about 60% water and is excellent for keeping skin looking at its best:

- Water aids digestion, absorption, circulation, creation of saliva, transportation of nutrients, and maintenance of body temperature.
- Your skin contains plenty of water and functions as a protective barrier to avert excess fluid loss.
- Dehydration makes your skin look more dry and wrinkled.
- When you are getting enough fluids, urine flows freely, is light in color and free of odor.
- When your body is not getting sufficient fluids, urine concentration, color and odor increases because the kidneys trap extra fluid for bodily functions.

The Institute of Medicine concluded that an adequate intake for men is roughly about 13 cups or 3 liters of total beverages a day. The ideal intake for women is about 9 cups 2.2 liters of total beverages a day. This should predominantly be water as this is the purest liquid and is perfect for keeping skin truly glowing.

Finally, I have included a number of other book's I've written that you may find useful on fitness and also a number of great diet books and other fitness books that are a great read. And be sure to review this book on Amazon!

Remember fitness and staying fit is about getting to know your body and only you can become the ultimate expert on that front!

So there we have it - you will be on your way to getting that amazing body - have a go, enjoy the workouts and be the change! Good luck!

This Book Could also assist you with your Fitness Goals:

Vegetarian Bodybuilding Nutrition: How To Crack The Muscle Building Success Code With Vegetarian Bodybuilding Nutrition